The Dairy Dilemma: Lactose Intolerance and Tolerance

How the Domestication of Cattle Changed Human Genetics and Culture

Thomas E. Sox, PhD

The Dairy Dilemma: Lactose Tolerance and Lactose
Intolerance

How the Domestication of Cattle Changed Human Genetics and
Culture

Front cover photo: Holstein cow, Keith Weller, USDA Agricultural Research
Service; back cover: Cows on Colorado Great Plains, Scott Bauer, USDA
Agricultural Research Service

ISBN: 9798687609210

Pondview Press

Ambler, PA

CONTENTS

1 INTRODUCTION

Although modern humans first appeared about 80,000 years ago, we developed agriculture, domesticated animals, and dairy foods much more recently. These new food sources have profoundly affected our culture and genetics. In particular, dairy products are now a large part of the diets of the people of many nations and cultural groups. For some, dairy products are the principal source of protein, a major contributor to total caloric intake, and a key source of some vitamins and minerals. This source of nutrition first appeared only about 8000 years ago, quite recent in human evolution. Before this, humans had only consumed milk by nursing during infancy, but the domestication of cattle, sheep, goats, and few other animals suddenly created an abundant source of milk and foods derived from milk. Groups of humans who transitioned from hunter-gatherer lifestyles to become herders and farmers made this emergence of dairy animals possible. The new dairy products provided excellent nutritional benefits and were available throughout most or all of the year. However, this new food source did present one substantial problem.

Prior to domestication of dairy animals, all humans lost the ability to digest lactose, the sugar in milk, at the time of weaning or shortly thereafter. The intestines of infants contained the lactase enzyme that breaks down lactose, but its production ceased during childhood. When older humans attempted to consume substantial amounts of milk, they likely experienced the well-known symptoms of lactose intolerance. The evolutionary processes that drove the emergence of modern humans provided a solution to this problem. Rare mutations that allowed adults to continue digesting lactose appeared among these early dairy consumers.

These mutations provided a poorly understood but very powerful reproductive benefit to these adult lactose digesters, and natural selection caused these mutations to become increasingly common among the descendants of these early milk consumers. Today, human societies vary greatly in the persistence of lactase into adulthood. In some regions, over 90% of adults continue to produce this enzyme; in contrast, in other populations virtually no adults have this capability.

This book first traces the story of human domestication of grazing animals, development of foods based on dairy, and the ensuing genetic changes that allowed geographically diverse populations to metabolize lactose throughout their lifetimes. Later chapters explore the diagnosis and treatment of lactose intolerance in detail, as well as the overall importance of dairy to the human diet.

This is unabashedly a science book, and it draws upon many scientific disciplines. The quest of the scientist is to develop objective information based on observation and experimentation, and to use this information to expand the understanding of our world. Essentially, science should be a search for truth. This is a difficult craft. In particular designing experiments to answer a specific question (or in science jargon, testing a hypothesis) is often challenging. Limitations in experimental design that result from resource constraints or simple flaws in logic or planning may diminish the strengths of conclusions that can be drawn from a scientific study. Often such issues encumber the human clinical trials discussed in this book. The author has attempted to note the limitations of these studies and to explain how they impact the strength of conclusions that can be drawn.

The objective interpretation of scientific information is a further challenge to people attempting to practice this trade or to write about science. Unfortunately, we live in a time in which scientific information is often not viewed objectively, and the strengths and weaknesses of information on a topic are not considered. Current debates over the existence of global warming and the safety of childhood vaccines are two dangerous examples of the twisting and distortion of what should be objective information. Unfortunately, this distortion of science has also sometimes penetrated into the realm of human responses to lactose, particularly the severity of symptoms of lactose intolerance and the capability of lactose intolerant individuals to consume lactose-containing foods without adverse symptoms. The author has attempted to present information in this area in an objective manner, and he presents both strengths and weaknesses of pertinent research. The reader may sometimes be disappointed that this book does not provide firm conclusions for some topics, but rather just points out the limited (or faulty) data available. The shortcomings in the available information simply do not permit a prudent person to draw strong conclusions (and this is very often the case in science). Words of equivocation such as "maybe" or "perhaps" appear often. This does not reflect indecisiveness by the author, but rather puts forward a frank assessment of the strength of the current science. Unfortunately, the trend to "weaponize" science to support various viewpoints has also extended to some of the topics in this book. These attempts to misrepresent science or draw strong conclusions from weak data are clearly noted.

Finally, this work is not intended to be just a self-help book for those who suffer from lactose intolerance. Several such books of varying quality are already available. This book differs in focusing on the science related to all aspects of lactose metabolism. Exaggerated claims and misinformation are, sadly, rampant in the field of lactose maldigestion and intolerance. In contrast, this book strives for an objective presentation. Lactose intolerant readers will find explanations of the science that causes this condition and the various remedies available, but the subject matter goes far beyond what is standard for self-help books. The topics presented will also appeal to those interested in recent human evolution and members of the nutrition community. The reader will gain an expansive knowledge about the long interaction of humanity with the milk sugar lactose, and develop a factual basis for dealing with this annoying condition of lactose intolerance that occurs in many of those who cannot digest this sugar.

2 THE BASICS OF LACTOSE, LACTASE, AND DAIRY

THE ROLE OF DAIRY IN CIVILIZATION

The domestication of dairy animals, particularly cattle, has profoundly shaped the development of many human societies over the last 8000 years. Dairying first began in a few locations, but has now spread to most habitable areas of the planet. Some modern societies consume vast amounts of milk and other dairy products. For example, in the United States, per capita fluid milk consumption in 2015 was 72 liters, or 19 gallons. The people of Finland and Ireland are world leaders in consuming milk, with per capita levels about 70% greater than in the US. Average annual consumption of cheese in the US is 16 kilograms, or about 35 pounds. Finland, Iceland, and France lead the world in cheese consumption; their citizens on average consume about 26 kilograms (57 pounds) each year.[1] For many individuals, dairy products are a major source of protein and account for a large portion of total caloric intake.

In contrast, people in some other regions consume almost no dairy, despite living in environments that are hospitable to dairy animals. These marked differences in dairy consumption are largely attributable to variations among individuals in their ability to digest lactose, the sugar in milk. In many individuals an inability to digest lactose causes some level of undesirable gastrointestinal effects, including diarrhea, flatulence, and cramping. Symptom severity may range from barely perceptible to truly acute. Among some ethnic groups, almost all individuals are able to digest the lactose in fluid milk without ill effects. In contrast, many people in other groups are afflicted with these symptoms after consuming dairy, an obvious indication of lactose intolerance. These tendencies to consume or not consume dairy products, and the ability to fully digest lactose, trace their origins back to shortly after some humans gradually gave up their hunter-gatherer lifestyles and settled into fixed agricultural communities or wandering bands of pastoral herders.

Thousands of years ago, humans in multiple locations began to maintain herds of cattle and other milk-producing animals. Dairying quickly became a key part of many farming and nomadic societies. Our journey traces this story of the domestication of cattle and other dairy animals, development of practices for converting milk into other foods, and the subsequent genetic changes in some humans that permitted them to digest lactose throughout their lifetime. This dairy revolution has led to a world population in which some people produce lactase throughout their lives. In contrast, for most of the world population the capability to produce lactase shuts down after the time of weaning, and they lack functional levels of lactase for the remainder of their lives. They may develop the symptoms of lactose intolerance after consuming dairy products, with symptom intensity based on the type and quantity of dairy product consumed. Fortunately, scientific advances in the last few decades have led to the appearance of products and regimens that allow the lactose intolerant to consume lactose-containing dairy without ill effects.

The author has been involved with lactose intolerance and its treatments for almost 30 years. He has watched the science related to this condition explode during this period, yielding a story that is unexpectedly rich and complex. Hopefully, the reader will share this excitement, and develop an appreciation of how a small molecule, lactose, and the human body's ability to produce the enzyme lactase have helped to shape our civilization.

As an entry point as well as background for the later detailed discussion, the following paragraphs present a few salient points for the impatient reader or browser.

LACTOSE INTOLERANCE IS NOT A DISEASE!

To begin with, the inability to metabolize lactose (commonly known as "lactose intolerance" or "lactose maldigestion") is certainly not a disease, nor generally cause for serious health concerns. In fact, the great majority (about 70-80%) of the world's adult population lacks the ability to digest lactose. Only certain individuals who are descended from some European, African, Central Asian, Indian Subcontinent and Mid-Eastern populations are able to fully digest dairy in adulthood. These populations generally share a common cultural background of domesticated dairy animals (primarily cattle, sheep, goats, water buffalo, and camels) along with a reliance on milk from these animals for a substantial portion of their nutrition. Although some other animals are locally important dairy sources, cattle are by far the greatest source of dairy products, and this book largely focuses on cattle. Chapter 3 traces their domestication, spread across the continents, and the resulting effects on human civilizations. Genetic changes, or mutations, allowing adults to digest lactose have appeared multiple times in these dairying populations. These mutations expanded rapidly in these populations because adult lactose digestion provided a strong natural selection. Chapter 4 tells the story of how some adult humans came to be genetically lactose tolerant.

In contrast to the diversity among adults in their ability to metabolize lactose, virtually all babies and young children can digest lactose. Nursing babies consume substantial amounts of lactose in the mother's milk. Human mother's milk contains about 7% lactose, and this lactose makes up 41% of the total calories in her milk. The ability to digest this lactose is thus crucial for the growth of the infant. Before the recent understanding of the science related to lactose digestion, the very rare babies born without the ability to digest lactose often died from diarrhea and malnutrition early in infancy.

WHAT IS LACTOSE, AND WHY IS IT PRESENT IN MILK?

Lactose is a sugar, and the major carbohydrate in milk. In contrast to the 7% level in human breast milk, cow's milk is about 5.4% lactose, and goat's milk is 4.1%. As noted, lactose provides a considerable portion of the calories in milk; protein and fat provide the rest.

Sugars are classified as either simple or complex. Simple sugars are small molecules containing five or six carbon atoms linked together in a row, with oxygen and hydrogen atoms attached to this carbon backbone. The combination, or chemical linking, of two or more simple sugar molecules forms complex sugars. Lactose is a disaccharide, a complex sugar composed of two simple sugars, glucose and galactose. Importantly, lactose is too large to be significantly absorbed through the walls of the healthy human small intestine. If it is not broken down into simple sugars in the small intestine, it reaches the colon intact, where its fermentation by the abundant microorganisms there causes symptoms such as gas, bloating, cramping, and flatulence that are so characteristic of lactose intolerance. In contrast, if effective levels of lactase are present in the small intestine, it releases glucose and galactose from lactose. These simple sugars are readily absorbed across the lining of the small intestine into the bloodstream. As they pass through the body via the bloodstream they are metabolized, providing the body with energy. The small intestine usually absorbs these simple sugars completely, and they do not cause lower gastrointestinal (GI) symptoms.

The reader may wonder why milk contains this disaccharide, lactose, instead of just the two simple sugars glucose and galactose. The answer to this is not entirely clear, but we do know that lactose is the principal sugar in the milk of almost all mammals, so this feature evolved well over 100 million years ago and is maintained in almost all mammals. Exceptions are the ancient egg-laying mammals such as the echidna and platypus of Australia. Instead of lactose, the milk of these animals contains carbohydrates that are more complex.[2] These animals are considered representative of the earliest mammals, essentially living fossils. It is unclear if these egg-laying mammals reflect the physiology of all early mammals, and in later mammals these milk carbohydrates were simplified to lactose. Alternatively, perhaps these surviving egg-laying mammals are just an evolutionary sideshow.

The mammary tissue produces lactose by linking two molecules of simple sugars. This process is complex, and consumes considerable energy that could have been used by the body for other purposes. The long evolutionary conservation of lactose despite this energy demand suggests that it serves some key role. One possibility relates to the osmotic strength of milk. "Osmotic strength" is a measure of the concentration of all the materials dissolved in a liquid. For example, honey, which is a concentrated solution of sugars that bees obtain from the nectar of flowers, has a very high osmotic strength. In contrast, pure water by definition has no osmotic strength. If milk contained free glucose and galactose instead of lactose, it would have a considerably higher osmotic strength. Consuming a large amount of something with high osmotic strength could cause fluids to be drawn into the intestine from the body, potentially triggering fluid loss and watery diarrhea. This could be a serious problem for a delicate infant. Production of a high osmotic strength fluid by the mammary glands might also pose physiological problems. Regardless of the reason, lactose appears to play an essential role in the nutrition of almost all young mammals.

As noted, the body uses the simple sugars glucose and galactose as energy sources. The situation with glucose is simple. It is the main carbohydrate fuel in humans, and virtually every cell of the body uses it readily. In contrast cells cannot use galactose directly as an energy source, and they must be first convert it into glucose by a series of enzymatic conversions. Rare genetic deficiencies in some humans block one of several enzymes involved in this conversion, and an alternative pathway converts the accumulated galactose into a compound known as galactitol. This gathers in the body to cause a disease known as galactosemia, which results in severe developmental issues in babies. The primary treatment, obviously, is to avoid breastfeeding and dairy products, since other foods do not contain appreciable amounts of galactose in an absorbable form. If not treated properly, galactosemia results in later neurological issues and speech impairment.[3] Fortunately, in people with normal galactose conversion pathways, dairy consumption does not result in galactitol accumulation.

WHAT IS LACTASE, AND WHY IS IT IMPORTANT?

The lactase enzyme is a protein that is able to break the chemical bond that links glucose and galactose to form lactose. The enzyme active site is highly specific, and only attacks this bond. Specific cells lining the small intestine produce it, and it remains bound to the surface of these cells. The lactase producing cells are located at the tips of small hair-like appendages in the intestinal lining known as villi. These villi are covered with even smaller protrusions known as microvilli, the location of lactase. Villi and microvilli immensely increase the surface area of the intestine, and they are the site of most absorption of nutrients from digested food. From the vantage point provided by these microvilli, lactase is exposed to the passing intestinal stream of partially digested foods or beverages, and it cleaves any lactose into simple sugars. Thus if an individual produces lactase, the lactose in dairy products is promptly broken down, and the resulting glucose and galactose are quickly absorbed. This process is highly efficient, and normally only a very small portion of passing lactose is not broken down. If an individual does not produce lactase, the intact lactose escapes digestion in the small intestine and enters into the colon, where the resident bacteria metabolize it. The accumulated lactose may also cause osmotic diarrhea, one of the well-known symptoms of lactose intolerance. In addition to these symptoms, the sufferer also loses most of the nutritional benefit of lactose, and possibly some of the benefit of dairy protein as well because of accelerated transit of the partially digested foods (known as "digesta") through the intestine. Chapter 7 covers the diagnosis of the symptoms of lactase non-persistence and lactose intolerance in detail.

Lactase is the most common name for this enzyme that cleaves lactose. However, in the scientific literature it is sometimes described by the awkward term "lactose-phlorizin hydrolase." Phlorizin is a compound found in a few foods, particularly very unripe apples. Trace amounts also occur in strawberries.[4] It consists of glucose attached to phloridzin, a flavonoid molecule. (Flavonoids are purportedly healthy compounds present in many fruits and vegetables.) Human lactase is capable of releasing glucose from phlorizin in addition to its better known role in digesting lactose. The enzyme apparently has two active sites, with the lactase cleavage site being distinct from the site that attacks phlorizin glycosides.[5] This may be an example of evolution using single proteins for multiple purposes. Phlorizin is a miniscule part of the human diet, and this separate enzyme activity seems to have no role in health or nutrition. More likely, this second enzyme activity is just a quirk of biology. Another frequent name for lactase is beta-galactosidase. This name is appealing to biochemists, because it is more descriptive of the specific reaction carried out by the enzyme. This term appears frequently in the scientific literature. The simple term "lactase" is used throughout the remainder of this text, but the reader should be aware of these other terminologies.

A FEW KEY DEFINITIONS RELATED TO LACTOSE DIGESTION

Before plunging into more detail in the following chapters, the reader will benefit from an understanding of a few terms related to human lactose metabolism and lactose intolerance. An understanding of these terms is key to grasping the subtleties of these topics. They appear frequently in the remainder of this book, and bookmarking this page may be helpful.

- "Lactose digestion" refers to the ability to produce amounts of lactase in the intestine that are sufficient to break down the lactose consumed in milk or dairy foods. This enzyme breaks lactose down into glucose and galactose, and thus lactose is "digested" by this intestinal enzyme.
- "Lactose maldigestion" occurs in the absence of sufficient amounts of intestinal lactase to break down the lactose in a normal serving of a dairy food, such as a glass of milk. The lack of enough lactase results in intact lactose being passed on to the colon, or large intestine. Lactose is "maldigested" because it is not broken down by a digestive enzyme, lactase. The term "malabsorber" is also used for this condition, since the absence of lactase prevents the absorption of the simple sugars comprising lactose.
- "Lactose tolerant" individuals have the ability to consume dairy products without the development of obvious symptoms. People who are lactose digesters are lactose tolerant. Importantly, a considerable portion of people who have lactose maldigestion (malabsorbers) are actually lactose tolerant. For them, lactose is not broken down in the small intestine, and it enters the colon intact. However, despite this they do not suffer the symptoms of lactose intolerance. The reasons for this are not entirely clear, but may reflect a bacterial balance in the colon that minimizes the symptoms resulting from lactose fermentation. Later chapters discuss this topic extensively.
- "Lactose intolerant" individuals are lactose maldigesters, who develop the characteristic symptoms of lactose intolerance (gas, bloating, cramping, and diarrhea) after consuming substantial amounts of high lactose dairy products. As noted, these symptoms result from the osmotic effects of unmetabolized lactose, as well as the gas produced during the fermentation of lactose by colon bacteria.

The above concepts of lactose digestion/maldigestion and lactose tolerance/intolerance are frequently confused in the media and in discussions of lactose and dairy. It is important to distinguish the subtle but significant distinctions between these terms, and to remember that lack of lactase (lactase non-persistence) makes an individual a lactose maldigester, but does not necessarily render that person lactose intolerant. The terms "tolerant" and "intolerant" refer to the perception of symptoms, and are conceptually distinct from the ability, or lack of ability, to digest lactose. These four bulleted terms are admittedly a little confusing, but you should take some time to master them before moving further into this book.

A continuing scientific dispute surrounds the amount of lactose that lactose maldigesters can consume without developing overt symptoms of lactose intolerance. Numerous clinical trials have addressed this issue, with huge discrepancies in results. Some investigators have found that lactose maldigesters can consume up to twelve ounces of milk without developing symptoms; others have found that only a couple of ounces of milk can cause severe symptoms in some individuals. This range of results may reflect details of the test (such as how lactose was consumed), the criteria used to diagnose lactose maldigestion, and how symptoms were assessed. The health and genetics of the individuals are likely involved as well. This controversy has also attracted the attention of various commercial interests, a situation that can lead to biased studies and generally bad science. Some individuals and organizations have viewed the public discourse about lactose intolerance as a threat to the dairy and food processing industries, since in their view this could discourage some individuals from consuming dairy. They would prefer to see this issue just go away; denying the existence of lactose intolerance symptoms is one way of achieving this end. On the other hand, some parties have claimed that miniscule intakes of lactose can trigger symptoms in some lactose intolerant individuals. This is hard to reconcile with what we know about GI physiology. Chapter 10 examines this controversy in more detail.

WHY ARE SOME PEOPLE LACTOSE INTOLERANT, AND OTHERS NOT?

The intestinal linings of all mammals stop producing lactase at about the time of normal weaning, except for some humans who are carriers of one of several mutations that allow lactase production over their entire lifespan. Although these genetic changes appeared only recently in human evolution, today about 20-30% of the world's population carry one of these mutations. Chapters 4 through 6 are devoted to the complex story of where these mutations appeared, and how they have spread through human populations. The term "lactase persistent" describes an individual who carries one of these mutations. Lactase persistent people generally do not develop symptoms after milk consumption. In contrast, those who do not carry one of these mutations may develop symptoms of lactose intolerance if they ingest milk after childhood. However, it is important to note that many people who do not produce lactase after childhood ("lactase non-persistent") are still able to consume moderate amounts of lactose in dairy products without suffering major symptoms. We will wrestle with this issue several times in later chapters. Even in people who are lactase persistent, the body may temporarily or permanently shut down intestinal lactase production because of disease or infection. This condition is known as secondary lactose intolerance, and is covered in Chapter 9.

It is important to note that when lactase production ceases during the childhood of a lactose intolerant person, that shutdown is irreversible. Most people who have studied biology in high school or college in the last 40 years learned about the lactose operon of *Escherichia coli* bacteria. The lactose operon is the classic example of gene regulation, and its discovery led to Nobel Prizes in Medicine in 1965 for Francois Jacob, Jacques Monod, and Andre Lwoff. Lactase is not usually present in *E. coli*. However, exposure of these bacteria to lactose causes them to produce lactase, in addition to several other enzymes. This bacterial lactase is known as an inducible enzyme because lactose exposure induces its production.[6] Any former biology students who still remember the lactose operon need to accept that this definitely does not apply to humans. Once the human gene for lactase shuts down, no amount of exposure to lactose, milk, or anything else, will cause it to regain its function. Chapter 4 explores why this shutdown is permanent.

WHAT IS THE ROLE OF ETHNICITY IN ADULT LACTOSE DIGESTION?

The presence of intestinal lactase and the ability to digest lactose in adulthood is largely based on an individual's genetics. Generally, individuals whose ancestors came from regions with strong dairy traditions are able to digest lactose. This includes a very large portion of people descended from northern

European stock. The portion of lactase-producing people is somewhat lower in populations from a number of other dairy backgrounds. These include southern and eastern Europe, the mid-East, northern India, and eastern and northern Africa (though a few African groups have very high levels of lactase persistence). In the remaining global populations, virtually all individuals are unable to produce lactase after childhood. This includes most of western Africa, most of East Asia, including China, and the original inhabitants of the Pacific islands, Australia, and the Americas.

ARE THERE OTHER FUNCTIONS FOR LACTOSE AND LACTASE IN HUMAN HEALTH?

Lactase serves a physiological function of converting lactose back into simple sugars that can be readily absorbed in the small intestine. However, there is speculation that on a higher level the duo of lactose and lactase may serve as a regulatory system for controlling the reproduction humans and other mammals. The Swiss scientist Harald Brüssow[7] has proposed a tantalizing but somewhat complicated theory that this pair evolved as a natural contraceptive process. In his view, a young animal's shutting down intestinal lactase production provides a signal to the mother's body that the appropriate time for another pregnancy has arrived. When a mother nurses an infant, hormonal changes that block ovulation are stimulated, and a mother generally is unlikely to become pregnant while nursing. (Readers take note: This process is too unpredictable to be a reliable contraception strategy.) When the infant's lactase levels begin to decrease, milk is no longer so palatable, and the young animal is stimulated to find other food sources. The end of nursing causes the mother's lactation to decline. This reverses the hormonal suppression of ovulation, and the mother is able to conceive again. In this theory, the duo of the milk sugar lactose and intestinal lactase (produced only during infancy until mutations to persistence appeared in some humans) are a mechanism for controlling pregnancy in mammals. In humans, this tends to provide a spacing of two to four years between births. Nursing puts strong demands on the nutritional and physiological health of the mother, and the nursing mother is not well-suited to bear the additional demands of a simultaneous pregnancy. Becoming pregnant while nursing could jeopardize the health of both infant and fetus as well as the mother. Nursing, and the cessation of lactase production by the weaning infant, provide a clever means for solving this problem. This theory by Brüssow is certainly provocative, and remains entirely in the realm of speculation.

WHAT TOOLS ARE AVAILABLE FOR DEALING WITH THE SYMPTOMS OF LACTOSE INTOLERANCE?

Many readers will explore this book in order to understand and manage the symptoms that they experience after dairy consumption. Learning about the physiology of this condition will help them to understand why their bodies sometimes negatively respond to dairy. A number of tools are available for managing this condition. One set is diagnostic tests to determine if GI symptoms are actually due to lactose malabsorption (i.e. failure to digest lactose), or if they are caused by an allergic response to milk or some more serious underlying medical problem. Chapter 7 describes these diagnostic tests. A second set of tools are products to help those sufferers trying to manage the symptoms of lactose intolerance. Chapter 11 covers these approaches, and the history of the medical understanding of lactose that led to their development. Remedies for lactose intolerance vary widely in effectiveness as well as the quantity and quality of scientific information that support them. Also repeated experiences of unpleasant and embarrassing lactose intolerance symptoms can induce continuing stress about dairy consumption in some individuals, and this stress may further exacerbate severity of the symptoms. Chapter 12 covers approaches to breaking this cycle of symptoms and stress.

The following chapters span many diverse fields of science. They target individuals with some knowledge of biological sciences, but most diligent readers will be able to understand the content. Endnote references are provided for those eager to explore the original literature, which provide much more detail as well as insights into the scientific sleuthing process. The author has intentionally emphasized references that are freely available in the public domain, and full text copies of many references are available through PubMed or Google Scholar® websites. Some chapters contain extensive technical material, particularly Chapter 4, which deals with the genetics of human lactase persistence and non-persistence. Unfortunately this subject matter cannot be readily simplified, and the author was not disposed to make this a textbook on molecular genetics. The complex information in Chapter 4 has been included in an attempt to make this book a comprehensive resource.

Let us begin with the story of how humans and cattle entered into a long-term relationship that has led to dairy foods representing a large portion of the diets of many people, driven genetic changes in humans, and even reshaped the landscape of much of the planet.

3 OUR DOMESTICATION AND ADULATION OF CATTLE

This chapter explores how the human relationship with milk-producing animals (mainly cattle) developed, and how the domestication of cattle in apparently just two locations preceded their spread over most of the habitable portions of our planet. This sets the stage for the next chapter, which describes how ruminant domestication has affected human evolution.

HUMANS SETTLING DOWN – THE DEVELOPMENT OF AGRICULTURE AND HERDING

For the last several million years the Earth has alternated sharply between periods of warmth and cold, driven by oscillations in its orbit around the Sun, and possibly variations in the intensity of the Sun. The cold periods have resulted in development of enormous glaciers in the cooler parts of the Northern Hemisphere, and at least twenty of these cycles of glaciation and subsequent melting have occurred. The drop in ocean levels caused by water trapped in the glaciers resulted in the joining of previously separate landmasses. Examples include a land bridge between Siberia and Alaska, and the present British Isles becoming part of the landmass of Europe. The gradual retreat of the most recent Ice Age glaciers about 13,000 years ago produced dramatic changes in the climate, geography, and environment of these northern areas. Lands previously covered by ice or grassy tundra turned into dense forests. Most of the large animals, including mammoths and mastodons, that had served as a food source for humans hunting in these northern areas also disappeared, likely because of both climate change and being pursued to extinction by these hunters. The fact that these animals had survived multiple previous Ice Age transitions (all of which occurred prior to evolution of modern humans) but perished in the most recent one strongly implies some human responsibility. Over the temperate regions of most of northern Europe and western Asia only a few large herbivores (plant eaters) remained, including the auroch, which was the ancestor of modern cattle; the wisent, a Eurasian species of bison; and the moose.

Some millennia after the glacial retreat, groups of humans began to abandon the hunter-gatherer lifestyles that our ancestors had lived for millions of years. Instead, they gradually began to cultivate plants and domesticate some of the wild animals they had previously hunted. These animals included a number of ruminant (cud-chewing) herbivores such as cattle, sheep, goats, and water buffalo. The use of milk from these animals as a food source developed soon after domestication. Cattle have had by far the greatest effects on human civilization, and this chapter will explore the domestication of cattle, their spread, and their wide-ranging effects on human cultures and societies. The development of a dairy culture was soon followed by the appearance of adult lactase persistence in some people in these societies. The next chapter presents the complex story of the genetic changes that caused humans to become lactase persistent. Together, these two chapters tell a story of how domestication of the auroch has affected the evolution of both cattle and humans.

This gradual transition from hunter-gatherer populations to a more fixed agricultural society centered on the cultivation of plants and the domestication of some animals began about 10,000 years ago. The era of hunter-gatherer cultures before the development of agriculture is known as the Paleolithic Period. The Mesolithic Period was a transitional epoch in which human cultures contained a combination of both hunter-gatherer and agricultural practices. This was followed by the Neolithic Period, which is associated with a full complement of related attributes including agriculture, domesticated animals, permanent houses and other structures, and complex pottery. The term "Neolithic Package" describes this group of cultural practices. These epochs are somewhat artificial distinctions created by anthropologists, and it is likely that human groups during these epochs pursued a wide variety of lifestyles, mixing many aspects of the Paleolithic and

Neolithic cultures. For example, some hunter-gatherer groups exploited areas with abundant fish or shellfish. These concentrated food resources allowed them to develop permanent settlements despite not farming or raising animals. Other groups likely incorporated some level of plant cultivation into their hunter-gatherer cultures, and perhaps changed their means of livelihood on a seasonal basis.

It is unclear whether this transition from the Paleolithic to Neolithic was driven by some superior benefits of this new lifestyle, or whether it was forced on struggling humans by declines in the resources essential to a hunter-gatherer existence (such as the extinctions of large game animals over much of the Northern Hemisphere). Regardless, this new lifestyle resulted in much higher population densities and the later emergence of villages and substantial towns based on trading, religion, and governance. This transition occurred at several locations in temperate and tropical climates, and two of these temperate areas are key to our story of the development of dairy. One site is the region known as the Fertile Crescent, which is a curved area beginning in modern Iraq, extending into portions of Turkey and Syria, and curving along the shores of the eastern Mediterranean. A second location is in the Indus Valley of modern Pakistan. In both these locations, the domestication of cattle, sheep, and goats soon followed the establishment of agriculture.

BENEFITS OF DOMESTICATING DAIRY ANIMALS

The development of animal husbandry by these early farmers may have provided a means for introducing more protein into a plant-based diet. Aside from serving as a food source, domesticated animals performed many other roles in these societies. In groups that farmed, these animals also provided a mechanism for converting agricultural waste such as hay and plant residues into protein, as well as providing manure that could serve as a fertilizer or fuel. Later domesticated animals provided traction for tilling the earth and hauling loads, particularly after the development of plows and wheeled carts. Animal body parts provided numerous resources, including horns and bones for use as tools, hides that could be tanned to provide leather, sinews for stitching, and stomachs for use as storage containers. A decline in the availability of large wild game perhaps made domestic animals even more important as a source of these raw materials.

Domesticated animals also provided highly visible and portable possessions. Today many herding cultures in various parts of Africa and Asia view cattle, goats, and sheep as a source of wealth, and these earlier societies may have similarly viewed these animals as a form of money. As we shall see later, these animals, particularly cattle, also took on broader cultural aspects. Early artwork in the Fertile Crescent demonstrates a prominent role for livestock in religious or cultural ceremonies. Some anthropologists have speculated that these cultures originally domesticated cattle for symbolic purposes, such as in rituals or religion.[8] Finally, when difficult times arose, they could use the animal herd as an emergency source of food.

The traditional view has long been that the development of agriculture and the domestication of animals, and humans' eventual settlement into fixed communities, was a great advancement for humanity. Certainly it was a prerequisite for the emergence of our current civilization. However, some have insightfully questioned whether this process was beneficial for the humans experiencing it.[9] Intense farming resulted in humans becoming dependent on just a few cultivated plants for their survival, and consequently crop failures could have had devastating impacts. Higher population densities associated with agriculture limited the ability to revert to a hunter-gatherer lifestyle, even if the famine-stricken individuals still retained the needed complex skills. In contrast, nomadic societies had a wider range of food resources, and could more easily relocate to areas with better resources.

Even in the absence of crop failures, agriculture seems to have provided poorer overall nutrition and health than the hunter-gatherer lifestyle, as evidenced by the decrease in stature of men and women during this transition. Analysis of bones recovered from Mesolithic and Neolithic burial sites in the Danube Valley showed that the average height of men and women decreased by about three and two inches, respectively, during this transition.[10] Women of this region did not again reach their average Mesolithic height again until the medieval period, and men's recovery was later still. There was also a major decline in dental health during this transition, with an increase in caries (cavities) that is characteristic of a high carbohydrate diet. Interestingly, skeletal remains from an early Neolithic cemetery in the Czech Republic indicated a higher incidence of caries in women than in men, possibly reflecting a higher carbohydrate diet.[11] Perhaps men had greater access to sources of animal protein and fat, with women relegated to a poorer diet high in carbohydrates.

Many other problems likely accompanied the transition to a sedentary agricultural lifestyle. The increasing population and crowding that accompanied a sedentary lifestyle permitted rapid spread of infectious diseases, which have devastating impacts in the absence of modern medicine. Densely populated communities allowed parasites and disease-carrying rodents to thrive. Human and animal feces may have contaminated water supplies, setting the stage our outbreaks of diarrheal disease. On a social level, a sedentary existence made the population more subject to taxation, enslavement, and capricious domination by government and religious elites. Social stratification led to a wealth-based mix of well-nourished and malnourished individuals. Animal domestication and dairying may have helped to alleviate at least the nutritional problems of these new societies, and this benefit may help account for the rapid spread of domesticated dairy animals.

Domestication of animals resulted in an intimate relationship with their keepers, as exemplified by chores such as milking, feeding, and manure removal. This resulted in human exposures to the microorganisms inhabiting these animals that were much more intense than would occur in just killing and eating wild animals. It is likely that these animals exposed humans to new diseases (and vice versa). Several recently emerged human infectious diseases, including smallpox and measles, are quite similar to diseases of cattle (cowpox and rinderpest, respectively). There is speculation that they evolved from diseases of cattle,[12] though there is scant information to support this view. Regardless, early humans may have acquired equally harmful diseases from their livestock. This would have driven natural selection for survival of humans who were more resistant to these diseases, or who readily developed immunity. As animal rearing spread and exposed naïve new populations to these animal-borne diseases, mortality may have reduced the ranks of the more susceptible people in these previously unexposed populations. This perhaps facilitated the spread and numerical dominance of the agriculturists and pastoralists who had already evolved resistance to these animal-derived diseases. Regardless of the cause, once these cultures combining agriculture and dairy animals developed they appear to have spread rapidly from their points of origin, displacing or incorporating existing populations.

THE RUMINANT STOMACH: THE KEY TO PRODUCTIVITY OF DAIRY ANIMALS

The animals domesticated in the Fertile Crescent and the Indus Valley were the precursors to our modern cattle, goats, and sheep. Other early societies domesticated additional grazing animals, including yaks, camels, water buffalo, and llamas. These animals are all ruminants; that is, they possess a stomach comprising four compartments, including the rumen. This complex stomach is crucial to both the nutrition of these animals and their ascent to prominence in human cultures. Fermentation of forage in the rumen allows them to increase greatly the nutritional value of their grazing diet. The ruminant stomach is one of nature's miracles to behold. It teems with a huge array of microorganisms, including bacteria, fungi and protozoa. In the warm, moist, oxygen-free environment of the rumen, these microorganisms convert otherwise indigestible plant matter into sugars and small compounds that can be absorbed from the animals' stomachs and intestines, providing a large portion of the total energy intake. Of particular importance is the ability of this complex microbial consortium to digest cellulose, the main component of most plant material. Cellulose is totally resistant to breakdown by human digestive enzymes, and humans excrete this dietary fiber with only slight degradation. In contrast, microbial fermentation in the rumen degrades cellulose into simple sugars that are further metabolized into nutrients that can be absorbed by the animal. These ruminants can thus thrive on plant materials that are inedible for humans, including dried grasses, leaves, tree branches, and almost any other plant material that they can chew.

The ruminant stomach makes these animals into very efficient producers of protein, and they convert biomass that is indigestible for most other animals into nutritious meat and milk. This unique digestive system is a largely unrecognized but important factor in the success of societies that exploited these animals.

Although early humans domesticated several species of ruminant grazing animals at various times and places, the focus of this discussion will largely be on cattle, since the great bulk of dairying throughout history is based on cattle. However, people in some regions long ago used milk from goats, sheep, camels, yaks, and water buffalo as a food source and these animals continue to play important roles in some societies.

THE EXTINCT AUROCH

Anthropologists have long sought to determine the earliest origin (or origins) of cattle domestication, and today the story is still incomplete. The now extinct auroch (*Bos primigenius)* is the ancestor of modern cattle. Before humans drove them to extinction, *Bos primigenius* and several closely related species had a huge geographic distribution, covering most of the non-polar Eurasian landmass ranging from the Atlantic to the Pacific Oceans, and extending into Africa. The auroch was an imposing animal with long, threatening horns. Bulls stood 60-70 inches high at the shoulder and weighed 1500-3000 pounds. Figure 1 depicts a reconstruction of an auroch bull based on a recovered skeleton.

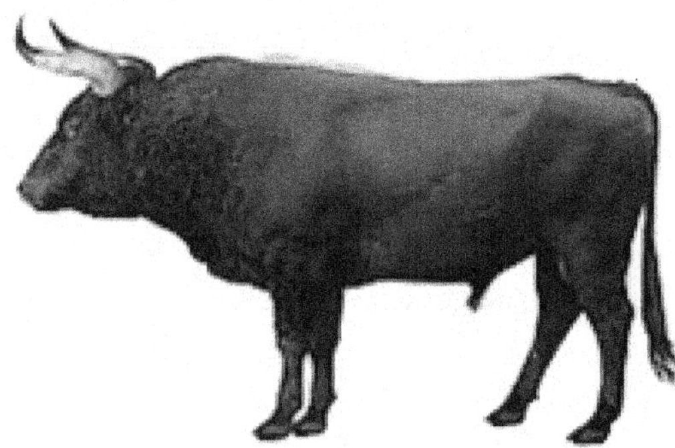

Figure 1: Restored auroch bull in the State Natural History Museum, Braunschweig Germany. Photo by Jaap Rouwenhorst, January 27, 2013. Reproduced under Digital Commons permission.

Aurochs are among the animals depicted in the famous drawings in the Lascaux Cave in southern France, which contains amazingly skilled art created about 26,000 years ago. One auroch depiction measures 17 feet long, the largest single drawing among hundreds in the cave system. The skilled painters often drew aurochs in association with wild horses. It is unclear if this reflected the two animals often being encountered together, or whether this pair had some cultural or spiritual significance.

Carvings in sandstone cliffs at Qurta, Egypt, overlooking the upper Nile valley of Nubia also prominently depict aurochs. These severely weathered rock carvings are around 15,000 to 16,000 years old. Aurochs are by far the most common figures, accounting for 136 of 179 recognized drawings on these cliffs.

Other depictions include hippopotami, gazelles, and humans. This artwork predates the appearance of domesticated cattle in Africa by many thousands of years, but it indicates that aurochs were already important to the culture of the pre-agricultural inhabitants of Qurta.[13]

Julius Caesar encountered aurochs while leading his soldiers through a vast forest in what is now Germany. He described them as "a little below an elephant in size, and of the appearance, shape, and color of a bull. Their strength is extraordinary; they spare neither man nor wild beast which they have espied. . . But not even when taken young can they be rendered familiar to men and tamed."[14] Fortunately, humans had tamed the auroch thousands of years before Caesar's commentary, and by his time cattle were much smaller and more docile than the auroch. Apparently Caesar did not recognize the auroch as the distant ancestor of Roman cattle.

DOMESTICATION OF THE AUROCH

One can wonder at how early humans domesticated these large and unruly beasts. Possibly calves of weaning age were captured and nurtured, thereby accepting some level of human control. An alternative hypothesis is that groups of humans and aurochs lived in close proximity, and the aurochs became so accustomed to humans that people began to actively manage the herds. This would be similar to the manner the Saami, or Laplanders, of northern Scandinavia use to manage herds of much smaller reindeer. They live in close relationship with the reindeer and selectively harvest animals for their use. However, they do not engage in traditional animal husbandry practices such selective breeding, feeding, or confinement.

The domestication of sheep, goats and pigs occurred in the Fertile Crescent and neighboring mountains slightly before auroch domestication. It is possible that the successful domestication of these much smaller animals provided an inspiration to early herders that they could also domesticate the auroch. The economic benefits of domesticating these smaller animals may have suggested the potential value of captive aurochs. A common assumption is that auroch domestication was motivated by the use of these animals as a source of meat. However, the widespread depiction of aurochs in paintings and carvings for thousands of years before domestication suggest that these animals may have had spiritual or cultural significance. This raises the possibility that symbolic importance of aurochs provided the original motivation for domestication. In addition, individuals with apparent control over these animals may have achieved a special social or power status, providing yet more motivation to tame and proliferate these animals.

Despite Caesar's commentary on their wildness, at least some of these aurochs could be tamed. Over time, these early herdsmen may have selected the most docile animals for expanding their herds, and they may have roasted the more unruly animals over the fire before they had a chance to reproduce. This continuous selection process led to the more gentle cattle of today (though bulls still deserve considerable respect). Domestication also led to a decrease in size of cattle. This again may have been a selection for animals that were easier to manage, or perhaps the smaller animals provided a benefit of consuming less forage during winters or dry seasons when they were largely dependent on food reserves accumulated by their masters. By the time of Julius Caesar, cattle were already appreciably smaller than their auroch ancestors. This decrease in size continued, and cattle reached their smallest size about 500 years ago. The specific genetic changes involved in the shrinking of aurochs into domesticated cattle are unknown, but are likely part of the broad package of genetic changes that humans selected into their herds. In the last couple of centuries, cattle breeds overall have become larger, and now are generally larger than cattle of Roman times. The recent increase in size of most cattle has been partly linked to a mutation that that arose about a thousand years ago in a gene known as PLAG1.[15] This gene is involved in regulation of insulin-like growth factor, which plays a role in the development of young animals. This mutation first appeared in Western Europe, and then rapidly spread to the cattle of many other regions. This suggests that increased size was then a trait highly prized by farmers, and their strong selection for such animals resulted in rapid spread of this mutation. Despite this recent trend toward increased size, modern cattle are still much smaller than their auroch ancestors.

In addition to size and temperament, the early herdsmen probably selected cows for breeding based on the amount and duration of their milk production. These various selection practices may have had other unintended consequences for cattle genetics. Often genes have multiple effects. The selection for one desirable trait is often accompanied by the appearance of other of less desirable traits linked to this gene. In other cases the desirable trait may also be accompanied by other traits that are neither beneficial nor harmful.

The tools of molecular genetics in combination with cattle bones recovered from early human settlements have provided a history of auroch domestication. Several lines of evidence, including the genetics of mitochondria, have contributed to this understanding. Mitochondria are small organelles found in basically every cell of higher organisms; they are the cell's energy generators. Each mitochondrion has its own single, very small chromosome that is distinct from the set of chromosomes found inside the nucleus of the cell. Fragments of mitochondrial DNA extracted from the bones of extinct aurochs have been sequenced to provide the complete DNA sequences of auroch mitochondria. Researchers at Trinity College in Dublin, Ireland, compared these auroch mitochondrial DNA sequences to modern cattle mitochondria to determine ancestry. They determined that the auroch was independently domesticated in at least two separate locations, the Fertile Crescent and the Indus Valley.[16] A distinct subspecies of auroch inhabited each region, and genetic analysis indicates that the two subspecies diverged from a common auroch ancestor about 250,000 years ago. Genetic differences between these lines provide tools for tracing the origin and spread of cattle derived from the respective auroch ancestors.

The Fertile Crescent gave rise to the breeds of cattle eventually raised in Europe and the Mid-East. These are known as the taurine breeds, for the Taurus Mountains that are near the putative area of domestication. Here archeologists estimate that auroch domestication occurred about 10,300 to 10,800 years ago. They have found remains of taurine cattle dating from about 7800 years ago in ancient human settlements in Anatolia, part of modern Turkey. These cattle were already smaller than their auroch ancestors. The decreased size of these animals (compared to the contemporary wild aurochs) is one indication that they were in fact domesticated, as smaller size often accompanies the domestication of animals. One of the earliest known sites of cattle domestication is Cayonu Tepesi, an ancient settlement on the Tigris River in southeastern Turkey. In addition to cattle, domestication of sheep, goats, and pigs occurred in this vicinity about this time or somewhat earlier. Based on analysis of bones excavated from the site, a decrease in size of mature animals of all four species quickly followed domestication[17] The decrease in size accompanying domestication is analogous to the general decrease in the size of modern dogs in comparison to the ancestral wolf.

Mitochondria are transmitted to the offspring only through the egg; sperm to do not contribute any mitochondria to the developing embryo. Thus mitochondrial DNA provides a way of tracking maternal ancestry. Different animals generally carry minor variations in their mitochondrial DNA sequences. The number of these variations present in a current population provides insight into the size of the original maternal founding population. The sequence data indicate that a relatively small number of females were involved in the Fertile Crescent domestication. Dr. Ruth Bollongino in Paris and her European associates sequenced mitochondria from cattle bones ranging from 1900 to 8000 years old collected from the Fertile Crescent.[18] They compared these sequences with those cattle currently raised in that region. This geographically limited sample avoided possible introgression (introduction of new genes by crossbreeding) from wild aurochs after the later geographic range expansion of domesticated cattle. They analyzed the sequence data by a complex statistical procedure to obtain an estimate of the likely number of female aurochs involved in the original Fertile Crescent domestication. Bollongino stated that "a large number (of females) would be expected if cattle domestication was a technologically straightforward and unexacting region-wide phenomenon, while a smaller number would be consistent with a more complex and challenging process" (p. 2101). Their analysis indicated that only about 80 females were involved in the Fertile Crescent domestication (95% confidence interval: 23-452). These findings do not determine whether a single domestication event occurred, or whether multiple domestications occurred in the Fertile Crescent. However, this analysis does indicate that domestication was a rare event, perhaps involving much difficulty or unique skills and resources. Perhaps local geography in some locations facilitated domestication. For example, humans may have trapped herds of aurochs in canyons or valleys from which they could not escape. Such captive populations may have become more accustomed to humans, and they provided the limited genetic stock that emerged as modern cattle. Domestication was likely a long process, involving slow genetic changes in both the appearance and behavior of the aurochs. Also, the continued development of cattle-managing skills by a small group of humans over centuries may have improved their ability to control cattle. These results suggest that domestication was not a process simultaneously carried out by many widespread groups in the

Fertile Crescent, but rather was the product of a relatively small group of unique individuals working over generations of both aurochs and humans.

As noted previously, a second domestication of cattle occurred in the Indus Valley region of the Indian subcontinent (hence the name "indicine" cattle). This domestication appears to have occurred slightly later than in the Fertile Crescent, but archeologists know less about this due to an incomplete fossil record and decreased research attention. The indicine cattle typically have a hump on their backs. They are more adapted to hot, dry environments, and they spread quickly spread through much of Southeast Asia. Taurine and indicine cattle can interbreed, yielding fertile offspring, and these cattle have intermixed multiple times during their histories. Land and sea trade between Europe and India dates back to at least the Roman Empire, and possibly this commerce included cattle. The later rise of the Islamic Empire facilitated a broader spread of indicine cattle, particularly westward and into Africa.

CHANGES IN CATTLE RESULTING FROM DOMESTICATION

The profound differences in appearance between aurochs and modern cattle breeds are the result of the numerous accumulated genetic changes. One way to identify these genetic changes is direct comparison of the chromosomal DNA of aurochs and modern cattle. Researchers at University College in Dublin, Ireland, sequenced DNA extracted from a 6700-year-old auroch humerus bone found deep in an English cave.[19] The bone predated the arrival of domestic cattle in the British Isles, and there was no possibility that ancestors of this auroch had crossbred with domestic cattle. Although these islands were part of the European landmass during the last Ice Age, rising seawaters had resulted in several thousand years of isolation for the British aurochs by the time this auroch bone found its way deep into a cave, perhaps in the jaws of a scavenger. This period of time was sufficient for the British aurochs to develop a genetically distinct population. By comparing the auroch humerus DNA sequence with the sequences of modern European cattle, the Irish researchers determined that current British and Irish cattle have more genetic similarity to this auroch than do other European cattle. This indicates that later wild aurochs in the British Isles bred with early domesticated cattle that reached these shores. Comparison of the 6700-year-old auroch and modern cattle DNA sequences revealed 263 changes in areas of functional DNA (i.e. DNA regions known to affect directly the phenotypes of cattle). These changes indicate that genes involved in neurobiology, growth, metabolism, and immune response are altered in modern cattle compared to aurochs. The neurobiology changes may have resulted in cattle that were tamer and more easily handled by their human masters. The changes in growth and metabolism may have resulted in animals that grew faster, and yielded more milk, or continued to produce milk for a longer time after calving. In addition, there were numerous changes in genes related to olfaction. Cats, dogs, pigs, and horses have also undergone changes in olfaction genes during their domestications. The significance that changes in sense of smell play in domestication are unclear, but the common prevalence suggests some function.

These initial domestications of cattle have been followed by thousands of years of cattle improvements (from a human perspective) by careful selection of breeding stock, and the development of breeds that can thrive in diverse and often adverse environments. Selective breeding has resulted in a plethora of cattle breeds around the world. Almost 1000 breeds are currently recognized, but the number is now declining due to the globalization and industrialization of the dairy and beef industries. Although we can compare DNA sequences of modern cattle breeds with the extinct auroch, fewer tools are available to indicate the chronology of how these changes have unfolded over the last 10,000 years or so. Domestication partly proceeded through a process of human-driven selection of useful or interesting traits. In addition, the new conditions of domestication and the novel environments where humans forced cattle to live likely affected their evolution. Compared to the wild aurochs, domesticated cattle may have suffered much more crowding and possibly consumed different food sources. Thus we can infer two categories of genetic changes following domestication. The first category includes the changes deliberately selected by pastoralists in their breeding efforts. These would have included traits such as docile behavior, milk production, horn size, and coat colors and patterns, as detailed in the following paragraphs. The second category is unselected changes that facilitated survival or reproduction of cattle under these new conditions. These may have included immune changes to make cattle more resilient in these new environments.

Domestication has had a very powerful effect on the morphology of cattle horns. Many current breeds show a dramatic decrease in horn size compared to the massive horns of aurochs, or an absence of horns (polling). Under the conditions of domestication, particularly crowding into confined areas, the large, spreading horns of the auroch would have been a hazard to other animals, as well as humans. It is not surprising that early pastoralists may have strived to develop cattle breeds with less ominous horns. However, it must be noted that today many breeds, including the aptly named Texas Longhorn, still sport imposing horns. The Longhorns are descended from the original cattle that Spaniards brought to the New World from Spain, beginning with the second voyage of Columbus. These escaped from captivity, and lived a feral existence in the arid lands of Mexico and the US Southwest for several centuries before becoming re-domesticated. The spreading horns may have provided a survival benefit to the feral animals, resulting in selection for large horns.

Current breeds of cattle vary immensely in color and color patterns. Dr. Imtiaz Randhawa and colleagues at the University of Sydney in Australia conducted a broad meta-analysis of the genetic changes in modern cattle breeds that contribute to the diversity of these traits.[20] The European auroch was a rather drab dark brown animal, likely an adaptation that made them hard to see in the dense forests that they inhabited. Occasional calves with mutations that caused different hide colors (such as brownish red, dark black, tan, and white) as well as spotted coats perhaps delighted early human pastoralists. They may have been intentionally selected this coloration in their herds, and unique coloration may have increased the value of these cattle in commerce. Today we know that coat color variations result from a number of gene mutations. The coat appearance of a specific animal is the result of interactions among several genes. For example, changes in a gene named KIT result in the white spots found on various breeds (similarly, variations in analogous KIT genes in other animals such as dogs are responsible for their white spots). Changes in the gene MCR1 alter the production of the pigment melanin found in skin and hair. Variations in this gene contribute to the various shades of black, brown, red, and yellow found in modern cattle breeds.

Another trait that humans may have selected was increased muscle size, which enhances meat yield. The hormone myostatin acts as a negative control that limits the development of muscle mass, and inactive variants (or mutations) of the myostatin gene result in greatly increased meat yield. Although this appears to be an appealing trait, animals that carry two inactive copies of myostatin are more prone to some diseases. Additionally, these cows generally have birth canals of reduced size, and their calves tend to be unusually large. Veterinarians frequently must deliver these calves by caesarian section, which greatly decreases the economic value of these animals.[21] It is unknown if more subtle variations in the myostatin gene or other genetic alterations entered into the development of cattle with more desirable meat properties.

Increased milk production is another obvious area of selection. This trait appears to be genetically complex, with changes in at least five distinct genes being involved. Our understanding of this area is poor, and additional research is needed given the economic importance.

The preceding discussion considered traits that have been actively selected by cattle breeders. A second category of unintentional changes includes alterations in immune function and resistance to disease. Newly domesticated cattle lived in confined spaces compared to the free-ranging nature of aurochs. Confinement may have increased the risks of infectious diseases, analogous to the higher disease exposure of humans as they settled into more crowded living conditions that accompanied the development of agriculture. Domesticated cattle were also exposed to diseases of humans, as well as the diseases of other domesticated animals that lived in close proximity, including goats, sheep, pigs, and dogs. European geneticists, after have examining genetic changes in modern European cattle populations, reported several alterations related to infectious diseases, including resistance to nematodes, mastitis, and bovine leukemia virus.[22] Some other observed genetic changes have broadly affected the bovine immune system, suggesting major shifts in immune function.

DISPERSION OF CATTLE TO EUROPE

After the initial domestication of cattle (and other ruminants) in some limited areas, they quickly became widely distributed in the Near East and adjoining regions. The island of Cyprus, which lies off the coast of Syria and Turkey, provides an example of this rapid dissemination. On a clear day it is visible from the Taurus Mountains of southern Turkey. Tectonic activity thrust this island up from the floor of the Mediterranean Sea and it was never part of continental Asia. Before humans intervened, it had just a few native mammals, limited mainly to now extinct pigmy elephants and hippopotami, and a native mouse. Humans began visiting and settling this island at least 12,000 years ago. Around 10,800 years ago, bones of several animals from the mainland suddenly appear in the ancient villages. These include pigs, goats, and cattle, with sheep arriving slightly later.[23] Interestingly, cats, foxes, and fallow deer also arrived at this time. Animal remains indicate that goats, pigs, and fallow deer quickly became feral and developed large wild populations, with extensive hunting by settlers. This provides a mixed picture of domestication and its reversal. Cattle appear to have remained domesticated and never developed large feral herds. In the remains of these early settlements, cattle bones are much less common than those of sheep or goats. Later, cattle disappeared completely from Cyprus until humans reintroduced them thousands of years later. This had led to speculation that these first cattle may have served a ritual function that was brought from the mainland by the early settlers, and after the island culture diverged from that of mainland Asia there was no longer a need for this ritual symbol with a huge appetite.[24]

The early presence of cattle on Cyprus demonstrates their rapid spread after domestication, even making a sea voyage from the continent to Cyprus. Cattle similarly spread quickly to other neighboring regions in Asia and Europe, and somewhat later into northern Africa. Geneticists have closely studied the spread of cattle through Europe, and this story is detailed below.

DNA sequencing of the Y chromosomes of modern cattle provide insights into the spread of taurine descendants through Europe. The Y chromosome is present in only males, and hence it provides a record of paternal ancestry, akin to how mitochondrial DNA traces maternal origins. Taurine (European) cattle are in a separate Y chromosome genetic group (or haplotype) from indicine (Indus Valley) cattle, confirming two different domestication events. Furthermore, based on DNA sequences the taurine Y haplotype itself can be subdivided into two major groups that differ in geographic distribution.[25] The Y1 group is found in northern and northwest Europe (including Ireland and Iceland), as well as the Iberian Peninsula. The Y2 group is more common in southern Europe. Both Y1 and Y2 haplotypes are still common in cattle of the Fertile Crescent region, further supporting this as a common site of domestication. Early farmers spread agriculture away from the Fertile Crescent, and their spread of cattle was closely linked to the expanding cultivation of plants, particularly grains such as wheat, barley, and oats. As noted before, this concurrent spread of domesticated plants and animals is part of the Neolithic package, which also include pottery. Anthropologists believe that the expansion of agriculture and the accompanying spread of cattle from the Fertile Crescent into Europe occurred via two routes. One, known as the Continental or Danubian route, spread up through the Danube Valley and into northern Europe. Agriculture and cattle spreading along this route reached Poland and Germany about 7500 years ago and entered Great Britain, Scandinavia, and Ireland about 1500 years later. This route may account for the current predominance of Y1 cattle in this region. Neither Y haplotype confers any known survival benefit, and the Danubian predominance of Y1 may just reflect a random effect in a small ancestral cattle population. A second southern route followed the coast of the Mediterranean and reached Greece about 9000 years ago, and Italy about 1000 years later. This route reflects the regions where Y2 cattle now predominate. Fossil DNA analyses indicate that all European aurochs were Y2, and the current Mediterranean predominance of Y2 mitochondria may partly reflect introgression of Y chromosomes from with wild auroch bulls. The following figure shows these two routes of cattle dispersion from southwest Asia into Europe.

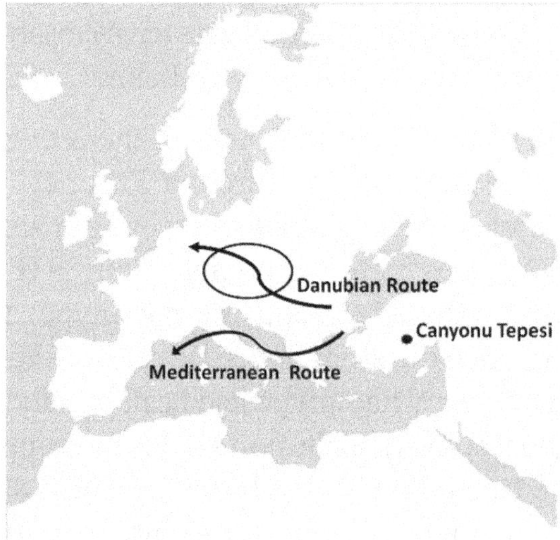

Figure 2: The likely routes of cattle spreading through Europe. Canyonu Tepesi is a site containing early evidence of cattle domestication. The oval indicates the likely area of emergence of a mutation that conferred adult lactase persistence, as discussed in the next chapter.

OTHER GEOGRAPHIC DISPERSIONS OF CATTLE: A MORE COMPLICATED STORY

Early farmers likely domesticated Indicine in the Indus Valley about 8000 years ago. Mitochondrial DNA sequences suggest later introgression from wild female aurochs in other areas of India, including the Ganges Valley. The indicine cattle continued to spread into Southeast Asia, and reached southeast China at least 2500 years ago.[26] They also reached island areas such as Indonesia and Philippines. Separately, taurine cattle also spread north into central Asia, and reached northern China about 4000-5000 years ago.

The idea of two discrete domestications of cattle (the Near East and Indus Valley) may be simplistic and is not uniformly accepted. For thousands of years after the first domestications, the wild auroch continued to roam much of Europe and perhaps Asia (the last auroch, a lonely female, died a natural death in a Polish forest in 1627). Since the ranges of domestic cattle and wild aurochs massively overlapped, it is likely that some interbreeding of aurochs and cattle continued to occur. Possibly European herders encouraged this, since it provided a way of introducing the beneficial traits of local aurochs into domestic cattle derived from aurochs that evolved in the much different environment of the Fertile Crescent. The presence of distinct auroch mitochondrial DNA in some modern cattle of southern Europe supports this hypothesis.[27] Since mitochondria are passed to the offspring solely via the egg, the presence of mitochondria with auroch DNA sequences in contemporary southern European cattle indicates that widespread interbreeding with auroch females may have once occurred.

Until recently, some scientists considered the high level of genetic diversity among cattle in North Africa to be evidence for a third separate domestication somewhere in this region. However, DNA from ancient North African cattle show great similarity to the early domesticated animals of the Fertile Crescent. Their genetic diversity may have originated by introgression from wild aurochs that still inhabited the area when the first herders arrived. Additionally, traits of these cattle were strongly influenced much later by zebu cattle introduced into Africa when this region came under Islamic influence. Today most scientists think that domestication only occurred in the Fertile Crescent and Indus Valley, and the broad genetic diversity found in North Africa is due to early breeding of taurine cattle with local auroch stocks, and the later introduction of indicine cattle.[28]

Finally, distinctive sequences of North African cattle are present in the DNA extracted from the bones of some early southern European cattle. This suggests that African cattle contributed to the genetics of this population, and indicates that there has long been transport of cattle across the Mediterranean. It is unclear how much of the spread of cattle along the European southern route was by land, and how much was by sea. However, the early presence of cattle remains on numerous Mediterranean islands indicates considerable transport by boat at an early date. The introduction of cattle to Cyprus very soon after domestication supports this. It is easy to imagine an early maritime trade in cattle between Africa and Europe that introduced African genetic influences.

This discussion of cattle distribution reflects the situation before the era of modern transportation, which has greatly accelerated the movement of cattle around the world. Today, on a global basis cattle genetics are very scrambled, with crossbreeding used to create varieties adapted to local conditions. For example, Indian zebu cattle were introduced into tropical areas such as Brazil for their heat tolerance, and herdsmen have crossed them with taurine cattle to combine the desirable traits of both groups.

RECREATING THE AUROCH?

As noted, the auroch has been extinct for several centuries. However, some cattle breeders have long been obsessed with resurrecting the auroch (or at least something resembling an auroch). Modern cattle still contain most of the DNA sequences of the extinct auroch (including auroch mitochondria), and identifiable genetic differences underlie the visually distinct varieties of cattle that exist today. Multiple efforts in Europe are attempting to interbreed existing cattle varieties to restore auroch characteristics, essentially weeding out the traits that many generations of herdsmen have selected into cattle breeds. The Heck brothers created the oldest auroch simulation, Heck cattle, in Germany in the 1920's. Enthusiasts still raise these cattle in Central Europe, and breeding is closely managed to emphasize auroch traits like size, horn shape, and coat color. This is a persistent interest by a group of dedicated cattle breeders, and a German book documents these efforts.[29] In the Czech Republic, a small herd of Heck cattle was released into "wilderness", the grounds of an abandoned Soviet military base, as a way of restoring a wild population. However, the Heck cattle are still much different from aurochs, with the bulls being much smaller, but stockier and less graceful than aurochs. One characteristic of Heck cattle that complicates their management is their aggressiveness (perhaps this trait does reflect a similarity to aurochs).

A consortium spearheaded by the University of Wageningen in the Netherlands is pursuing a separate more science-based auroch reconstruction. This program is using an approach based on DNA sequence data on current European cattle breeds, and the full DNA sequences obtained from bones of extinct aurochs. The goal is to cross existing cattle possessing specific wild-type auroch genes to create animals with increasing genetic similarity to aurochs. This program only began in 2008, but the ambitious goal is to have auroch-like animals ready for release into the wild shortly after 2025.[30] Perhaps someday herds of these auroch imposters will roam wilderness sanctuaries of Europe and Asia.

HUMAN ADULATION OF CATTLE

Domesticated cattle, particularly bulls, figured prominently in many early religions. As noted earlier, some scientists have speculated that the original domestication of cattle was related to their symbolic or ritual significance, rather than their economic value. The ancient Egyptians worshipped a number of animal gods with Apis, the bull, being most prominent. Apis represented both valor in war and fertility (impressively, one bull can readily impregnate a herd of 20 or more cows). In Memphis, a cult focused on individual bulls that they selected as sacred animals. The anointed Apis bull inhabited posh accommodations, received the best food, and had a harem of cows for entertainment. The bull's mother also received royal treatment.

Adherents believed that the Apis bull was able to foresee the future, and attendant priests carefully observed its behavior for hints at divining the future. There was a belief that young boys who smelled the Apis bull's exhaled breath would also develop powers of predicting the future. When an Apis bull died, there was a period of public mourning, with the carcass embalmed and entombed in a granite sarcophagus.

When the Jews fled Egypt and entered the Sinai, they faced idolatry in the form of cattle worship. Seeking spiritual guidance, Moses withdrew to Mount Sinai for forty days and nights, causing the Jews to become impatient and religiously restless. They asked Aaron to make gods for them to worship. To oblige, Aaron collected the gold jewelry from the people and melted it into the form of a golden calf. Aaron built an altar in front of the calf, and the people brought offerings and sacrifices. Moses returned to witness this astonishing spectacle. He became so angry that he broke the inscribed stone tablets he had carried down from the mountain. It is unclear if this worship of the golden calf represented a tradition that the Jews had recalled from the culture of Egypt, or whether it was an adoption of practices of Canaanites who already inhabited the region.[31]

A deep respect for cattle also permeates the Indian subcontinent. The term "sacred cow" derives from the Hindu adulation of cattle, and reflects the belief among many Hindus that this animal is sacred. Hinduism is one of the world's oldest religions, tracing its roots back more than 3000 years. However, the sacredness of cows appears to have developed more recently. Early Hindu texts in fact did not ban the killing of cattle; instead they could be sacrificed in rituals, and consumed in accompanying feasts. By 1800 years ago, Hindu beliefs had changed. Cattle were now to be venerated, and abuse or slaughter was prohibited. The veneration of cattle increased after the Islamic invasion of India, possibly as a means of mental resistance against the beef-eating Muslims.

India is the world's largest producer of milk. Although dairy cows are nutritionally important in India, water buffalos provide greater total milk production (and a milk much higher in butterfat and protein). The greater economic benefit of cattle in India in the past may have been in the use of oxen (castrated bulls) to till land. There is speculation that the Hindu prohibition against cattle slaughter is underlain by an economic rationale. Traditional Indian agriculture was dependent upon the annual monsoon rains, which have erratic arrivals and occasionally fail completely. This led to periodic widespread famine distress for both humans and animals. Forbidding slaughter helped insure that farmers would not use draft animals for food during famine, and oxen and cows capable of producing new draft animals would still be widely available when the rains finally did return. Thus the religious standing of cattle could be regarded as a societal form of disaster insurance.[32]

THE ORIGINS OF DAIRY

Domestication of ruminants obviously involved raising new generations of animals, and lactating cows (as well as ewes and does) became common. The ready availability of milk provided a new source of nutrition. It is unclear how extensively these early pastoralists exploited milk from lactating cows, but archeological evidence indicates that humans in areas around the Fertile Crescent were milking cows shortly after domestication.

Chemical analyses of pottery fragments have provided insights into the first human uses of cow's milk. Dairy milk fat contains fatty acids (the major component of milkfat) that differ from those found in the fat of beef. Specifically, these are unsaturated fatty acids, in contrast to the predominantly saturated fats in meat. Scientists have developed methods for detecting the presence of these milk-specific fat residues in ancient pottery fragments. A report authored by Dr. Richard Evershed at the University of Bristol in the United Kingdom and 21 coinvestigators from seven countries describes a massive effort to trace the origins of dairy.[33] Briefly, researchers thoroughly clean the surface of a pottery fragment to remove any modern contaminants, and grind the clean fragment to a powder. They stir this powder in a solvent mixture that dissolves any fatty acids that had seeped into the pottery thousands of years ago. These fatty acid residues are concentrated and identified by gas chromatography and mass spectrometry. A comprehensive analysis of 2200 pottery fragments collected from 23 sites in the Near East and southeastern Europe indicated the widespread presence of dairy fat residues in pottery samples from 5000 to 7000 years old. Thus the oldest traces of dairy fat on pottery residues are relatively soon after the domestication of cattle in the Fertile Crescent, indicating that humans quickly exploited this new food source. This research also determined that in some of the pottery fragments the dairy fat had undergone structural changes indicative of heat exposure. This indicates that Neolithic farmers quickly utilized dairy products in cooking.

Corroborating evidence for an early use of milk from domesticated cattle comes from an unlikely source, human dental calculus. Dental plaque is a deposit of bacteria and their metabolic products on the surface of teeth. Salivary proteins and remnants of food also become trapped in the plaque. This plaque gradually becomes mineralized to form a hard substance on the tooth surface known as calculus. Anyone who has had a dental prophylaxis is quite aware of how strongly calculus adheres to teeth. Calculus is very resistant to degradation, and remnants of it are still present on the teeth of humans who perished thousands of years ago.

Using an analytical technique known as tandem mass spectrometry, an international collaboration of researchers developed techniques for extracting proteins from ancient dental calculus and determining their identities.[34] Beta-lactoglobulin, a major protein in cow's milk, accumulates in the dental plaque of dairy consumers. Dr. Matthew Collins at the University of York in Great Britain led a team of researchers from six countries in using this technique to analyze plaque samples from human remains found in numerous locations in central and Western Europe. Beta-lactoglobulin was found in human dental samples up to 5000 years old collected in Denmark, Hungary, Germany, and Italy, independently confirming that consumption of dairy products was already widespread at that time.

These pioneering herders or farmers faced challenges in exploiting this new food. First, at that time virtually all adults were lactase deficient (and hence potentially lactose intolerant). Ingestion of significant amounts of liquid milk could have triggered the characteristic symptoms of lactose intolerance. Second, raw milk spoils quickly in non-hygienic conditions in relatively warm climates. Quickly processing the milk could have been partly avoided spoilage problems. The dairymen may have separated fat from milk to form butter, a calorie-dense food relatively resistant to spoilage. They may have intentionally fermented milk to form yogurt or kefir-like foods. These tend to have somewhat lower lactose levels, and contain bacteria capable of further degrading lactose after human consumption. Finally, they may have processed milk into cheese, a long shelf life food that could be stored for many months in cooler climates. Some of the pottery fragments containing dairy fat mentioned above were from pots that were perforated with many small holes. The perforated pots are similar to some strainers currently used to separate curds (precipitated dairy protein) from the whey liquid, which contains most of the lactose from the original milk.[35] This separation is an early step in cheese making. Pastoralists' development of these strainers suggests an early emergence of cheese-making technology, providing a portable food that was stable in the absence of refrigeration. Polish archeologists have excavated numerous strainer fragments, and the extrapolated shapes and sizes of some of these vessels are presented in Figure 3.

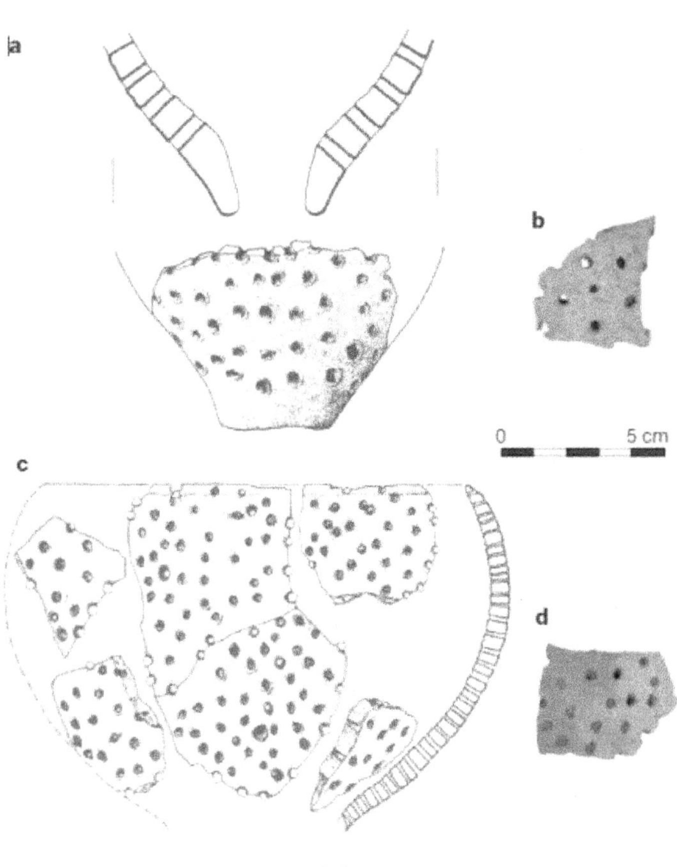

Figure 3: Strainer fragments excavated from the Kuyavia region of Poland; a and b are from the Brezseść site; c and d are from the Smólsk site. Reproduced with gracious permission from R. Grygiel, Museum of Archeology and Ethnography, Lódź, Poland.[36]

One downside of cheese making is that much of milk's nutritional value is lost. During cheese curd formation, some of the whey protein (a substantial portion of the total protein content) remains in solution, and is lost. Also, the milk sugar lactose, which accounts for another large portion of the overall caloric value, is largely lost.

Consumption of fresh milk offered one way of preserving the full nutritional value. As noted, genetic evidence indicates that adult humans prior to, and just after, the first domestication of cattle were lactase deficient.[37] They likely would not have been able to tolerate significant milk consumption. However, all young children could freely consume milk because functional levels of lactase were still present in their intestines. There is evidence that children even consumed very milk directly from the cow. A figure from an Egyptian tomb from the Fifth Dynasty (about 4300-4400 years before the present) shows a child and calf both suckling a cow.[38] Similarly, poorly dated primitive rock drawings in the Sahara Desert of present day Libya also show small human figures (presumably children) drinking from the udder of a cow.[39] This consumption of very fresh milk would have provided valuable nutrition for children, and the milk may have been safer than polluted water sources. This may have been key to survival of these children into adulthood, and could have reinforced the social value of dairy animals.

DISPERSION OF CATTLE AND DAIRYING

In Europe, the spread of domestic cattle closely accompanied the expansion of agriculture; this is part of the previously mentioned Neolithic Package. This was not the case in other areas. In Africa, early herding cultures (similar to some of those of the present) engaged in little or no agriculture likely because of the arid climate. In addition, in other regions, particularly the New World, agriculture-based societies developed without development of dairying practices. The few ruminant mammals domesticated in the new world, such as llamas and alpacas, may not have been suitable for dairying. Similarly, the Chinese developed a complex agriculture-based civilization that did not include a significant dairy tradition. Cattle reached China only long after its agricultural system was well established. Thus the almost simultaneous development of agriculture and domestication of cattle in the Fertile Crescent and Indus Valley may reflect a specific response to the unique resources available.

Once domestication of cattle had occurred, humans over a wide geographic area were soon maintaining their own herds. It is somewhat unclear whether this spread occurred through the increase in number and geographic expansion of the people in these early herding societies, or whether adjacent populations adapted the skills needed to maintain cattle animals. Genetic analysis of DNA from bones of humans who perished thousands of years ago in Northern Europe suggest that people migrating into the area spread farming and animal husbandry, rather than earlier residents adapting these practices. Thus, the spreading agriculturalists largely displaced the hunter-gatherer peoples that had previously inhabited this area. It is unclear whether these earlier residents disappeared without a trace, or whether they became assimilated into the numerically dominant agricultural population.

As noted, cattle herding was widespread in Europe, Asia, and North Africa by at least 5000 years ago. Cattle spread over the remaining parts of the world during the period of European colonialism and expansion. Social and environmental effects accompanied widespread cattle raising. For example, by 1870 over 13 million cattle roamed over the Pampas of Argentina, and cattle products were that nation's primary export.[40] Cattle were similarly introduced successfully into many areas of North America and Australia.

On the northern edge of human occupation, the Norse introduced cattle into Iceland and eventually Greenland. Remains at ancient farmsteads in Greenland indicate that most farms had at least a few cattle, and the estate of a bishop had barns capable of housing 100 animals. These Norse outposts also raised sheep, goats, and horses. One can imagine the spectacle of Norsemen ferrying cattle and horses across the stormy North Atlantic in open boats (perhaps they transported young animals to reduce the weight of the live cargo and the feed needed during the voyage). After several centuries of Norse settlements in Greenland, a period of unusual cold (The Little Ice Age) reduced the amount of summer forage that could be dried and stored to feed livestock during the long winter months. The decline of cattle and dairying may have been a major contributor to the shrinkage and eventual abandonment of the Greenland settlements around 1450.[41] In addition, walrus tusks comprised much of the commerce from Greenland to Europe, where craftsmen carved them into numerous items. At this time, the much larger tusks of African elephants were becoming more common in Europe, and this may have undermined the economics of the walrus tusk trade and the overall financial viability of the Greenland settlements.

DEVELOPMENT OF MILKING

After giving birth a cow freshens, or starts producing milk and keeps producing milk until or after weaning the calf. The challenges for early dairymen were to collect milk without harming the growth of the calf, and to prolong the period of lactation, particularly after they weaned the calf or slaughtered it (a likely fate for surplus male calves).

Even after they weaned the calf, it may still have been important to milk production in these early cattle. The milk ejection reflex initiates the release of milk in lactating cows; this reflex is the result of increased blood levels of oxytocin. Oxytocin is a hormone with numerous physiological effects, many of them involving a sense of contentment or well-being. The sight of her calf, and the initiation of nursing, triggers oxytocin release in the cow's brain, allowing milk to flow. Even today, some animal husbandry practices involve keeping the calf after weaning, instead of slaughtering or selling it. The calf is presented to the mother at each milking to stimulate the flow of milk. Variations of this approach include presenting another calf, or even the skin of the cow's own slaughtered calf draped over a child or an appropriate stand. For word lovers, "tulchan" is a word for this fake calf.

Little is known about the ease (or difficulty) of milking the recently domesticated cattle of 6000-7000 years ago, the time of the earliest evidence of dairying. These early dairymen may have selectively bred cows that they could easily milk, possibly resulting in selection of gene variants related to the milk ejection reflex. In addition, sufficient docility to allow milking was essential.

Triggering milk release from the lactating cow was apparently a common challenge for early dairymen, particularly if the calf were no longer available (it may have died, or they may have eaten it). Several rock carvings in the Libyan Desert dating from about 3000 years ago appear to depict efforts to persuade cows to release milk. In these drawings, one individual lifts the cow's tail vertically with one hand, while placing his or her mouth on the animal's vulva, while a second person is in a position to milk the cow.[42] Carved panels from Sumeria from about 4500 years ago contain similar depictions of humans with their mouths placed on the private parts of cows. This artwork depicts a widespread practice known as "insufflation." This occurs in various forms; perhaps the simplest is that depicted in these carvings. With the cow's tail lifted out of the way, the mouth is placed over the vulva, and air is blown in forcefully. The vulva may be quickly sealed shut with the free hand, maintaining the inflation of the vagina and uterus. This somehow causes the cow to release more milk, but it is not clear if the cow finds this pleasant or irritating. In some pastoral societies, a reed or hollow bone was inserted into the vagina, and someone blew air through this tube. A more invasive approach to stimulate milk release was to thrust the hand and arm up to the elbow into the cow's uterus.

Insufflation has long persisted as a dairying practice. In 1681 Thomas Dineley, a visiting Englishman, described a practice used by dairymen in Ireland: "when milk doth not come freely [. . .] with their mouths to blow in as wind as they can, with which doing they many times come off with a shitten nose."[43]

In India, the process is known as "phooka." Gandhi viewed this process as cruel to animals, and this was a basis for his refusal to consume dairy products. In his autobiography, he stated: "Religious consideration had been predominant in the giving up of milk. I had before me a picture of the wicked processes [phooka] that govals in Calcutta adopted to extract the last drop of milk from their cows and buffaloes."[44] Subsequently, animal cruelty laws barred this practice in India, with penalties of a fine of up to 1000 rupees, up to two years in prison, and forfeiture of the animal to the government.[45]

The pioneering British anthropologist Edward Evans-Pritchard documented insufflation among the Nuer people of the Upper Nile in 1930's. The following figure is his relevant photograph from 1935. In addition to the individual practicing insufflation behind the cow, also note in the foreground a fake calf (tulchan) used to trigger milk release.[46] Insufflation continues in some parts of the world, as a YouTube® search of "phooka" or "cow blowing" will graphically demonstrate.

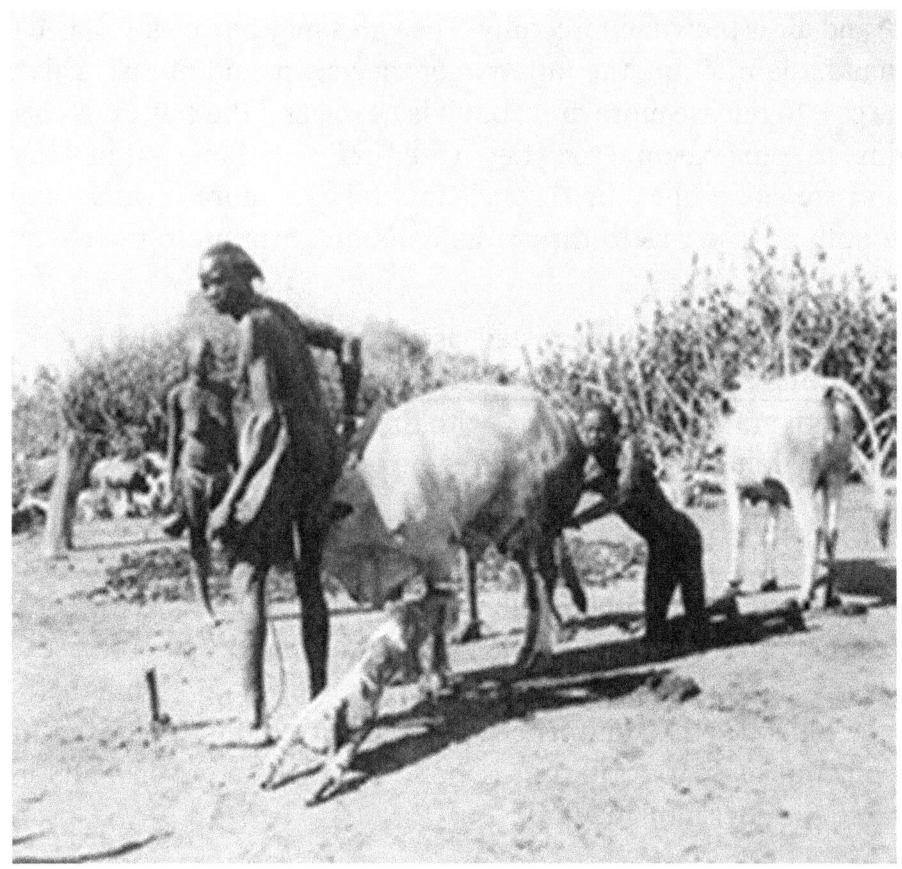

Figure 4: Insufflation in a Nuer dairy herd. Original photo by Edward Evans-Pritchard, about 1932. Copyright Pitts Rivers Museum, University of Oxford, Accession Number 198:355:447:2.

CATTLE RIVAL HUMANS IN GLOBAL DOMINANCE

As discussed earlier, the domestication of cattle was followed by humans dispersing them to almost all inhabited regions of the Earth. A large part of the global landscape, ranging from lush fields deep in grass to sparse deserts, is dedicated by grazing areas for cattle. Clearing of land for pastures has led to destruction of vast areas of tropical forest, including parts of the Amazon basin. Farmers plant other lands with crops such as corn, soybeans, and alfalfa that are used to feed these animals. Today a vast number of cattle inhabit the planet. Agricultural statistics from the Food and Agriculture Organization (FAO), a United Nations agency, track the populations of cattle of every nation.[47] According to 2014 data (the most recent available) India had the world's largest cattle population, 187 million; it also had 110 million water buffalo. The leading status of India is not surprising given the religious and cultural significance of cattle (and the fairly high incidence of lactase persistence). China was second, with 118 million. This is unexpected given the high incidence of lactase non-persistence and the small amount of arable land in proportion to the population. In third place with 88 million cattle is the United States, where cattle pastures are common in most states and both dairy and beef consumption are high. Even Greenland, where Vikings introduced cattle that disappeared during the Norse abandonment in the Little Ice Age, currently has about 15 cattle. In total, the planet supports about 1.6 billion cattle. These data are based on statistics reported by individual countries, or estimates developed by FAO, so these numbers may be somewhat inaccurate or exaggerated. However, given the relative size of humans and cattle, the total weight of cattle on the face of the planet is probably greater than the total weight of the Earth's 7 billion human inhabitants. As a broader sign of how humans have altered the planet's biodiversity, the combined weight of all domesticated animals is about 30 times the weight of all wild mammals ranging from mice to elephants that currently roam the earth's surface.[48]

The FAO data do not provide a separate analysis of the number of dairy cattle (this is a somewhat artificial distinction in many cultures). However, FAO does track milk production from dairy cattle. The United States is the world's leading milk producer, with 93 million metric tons produced in 2014. On a per capita basis, this equates to about 640 pounds of milk for every person in the United States (though many dairy products are exported). India comes in second at 66 million tons, showing the comparatively low productivity of Indian cattle. China was the world's third largest dairy producer at 38 million tons. On a per capita basis, dairy production in China in only about 10% of American production.

Much of the world's population is involved is this dairy enterprise. IFCN, a German dairy industry analysis organization, estimated that about one billion people live on dairy farms. Overall, the average dairy "herd" on these farms contains three or fewer cattle. This is in contrast to US factory dairy farms, which may contain thousands of cows.[49]

The immense number of cattle on the planet exert a huge environmental impact. The FAO estimated that the production of milk, including its processing and delivery, accounts for 2.7% of global greenhouse gas emissions.[50] Ruminant livestock, mainly cattle, account for 17% of the worldwide emissions of the powerful greenhouse gas methane. However, the human population needs to eat, and any other approach to providing people with protein and nutrient rich foods would also likely affect these emissions.

We have just explored the domestications of cattle, the development of dairying, and the spread of this culture across Europe, Asia, and Africa. The development of dairy set the stage for the multiple occurrences of human genetic changes that permitted adult humans to fully digest lactose. The next chapter presents the complex story of these changes.

4 THE GENETICS OF LACTASE PERSISTENCE

SIGNIFICANCE OF DAIRY ANIMALS AND LACTASE PERSISTENCE

Although cattle provided many benefits (including an obvious and portable source of wealth), milk and milk products quickly took on a role in the nutrition of most cattle-rearing societies. This development of a dairy culture resulted in the lactating cow becoming a continuing source of sustenance, in comparison to slaughter that would provide food for just a brief period and result in the destruction of an economically valuable asset. The human adults of these first dairy societies were likely limited in their ability to consume milk without experiencing unpleasant symptoms arising from the lactose content. Consequently much of the milk collected may have been processed into more stable foods such as cheese and butter, or fermented into lower lactose products. However, the substantial source of calories provided by lactose was largely lost from these foods. Continued production of lactase into adulthood (lactase persistence) would have conferred a significant nutritional benefit.

In all mammals the small intestine produces lactase from birth until about the age of weaning, after which the levels irreversibly decline (except in lactase persistent humans). This chapter focuses on the genetic changes that cause some humans to be lactase persistent, thus continuing to produce lactase throughout their lifespans.

Just as the domestication of cattle occurred in multiple regions, human genetic changes resulting in adult lactase persistence appeared several times in different locations. We know this from the record provided by the human genome, our set of 46 chromosomes as well as the separate mitochondrial DNA. The DNA sequences of individuals reveal a genetic history of their ancestry. Sequencing DNA samples from multiple diverse populations of lactase persistent people has revealed several different mutations (or alleles) that confer adult lactase persistence. In each of these populations, initially one ancestor was born with a spontaneous mutation that allowed lactose digestion after childhood. This adult lactase persistence resulted in a selective advantage for this individual if he or she were part of dairy consuming culture; later we speculate on the specific potential advantages. Due to the ability to digest lactose, this ancestor was somewhat more successful in surviving to adulthood and raising children than other members of the group. This individual thus passed this highly desirable new allele to his or her more numerous progeny, and natural selection in a milk-consuming society ensured that the allele became progressively more prominent in the population with each succeeding generation. Geneticists have used the human DNA record to develop a fascinating story of the history and spread of these lactase persistence alleles.

A BRIEF PRIMER ON GENETICS

Before exploring in detail the origins of lactase persistence, we must take a brief detour into human genetics for some essential background. The following presentation is admittedly cursory and deletes many of the intricacies of a complex process. Four molecules known as "nucleotide bases" are the building blocks of DNA; these are adenine, cytosine, guanine, and thymidine. DNA is made of two paired chains consisting of alternating ribose (a sugar) and phosphate groups; the nucleotide bases are attached to sides of these chains. Nucleotide bases on the opposing strands are attracted to each other through weak hydrogen bonds. These bonds only allow some specific pairings to occur – adenine and thymidine on opposing chains always pair together, and similarly cytosine and guanosine always pair. These weak bonds between specific nucleotide bases are the "glue" that holds the two strands of DNA together, and almost all DNA in the cell is in this double-stranded configuration. Thermodynamic forces cause the double strands to twist slightly to form a spiral, giving rise to the famous DNA double helix that James Watson, Francis Crick, and Rosalind Franklin first inferred from X-ray crystallography images in the early 1950's.

The sequence of these four bases in the DNA strand encodes all of the vast information in the human genome, similar to the binary system of zeros and ones that encodes all information in computers. These four DNA bases can occur in virtually any sequence in a molecule of DNA. Linear units of three bases make up the genetic code. Each three base sequence, such as adenine-guanine-cytosine (or AGC) is known as a codon. Most codons encode one of the 21 amino acids that are the building blocks of proteins, thus allowing translation of DNA sequences into the amino acid sequences that make up proteins. Sixty-four possible codons exist, based on all possible triplet combinations of these four bases (4x4x4). The genetic code is redundant, and some amino acids are encoded by multiple codons. Other specific codons establish the reading frame. This is the specific point in the sequence where translation of codons into the amino acid sequence of a protein begins. This prevents random reading of the base pair sequence, and ensures that the complex cellular machinery that translates sequence information into proteins reads this in a specific regulated manner. Similarly other codons serve as termination signals, stopping this translation process.

DNA in the cell nucleus is a storage device for genetic information, and is not the actual tool that is used to translate this information into proteins. Messenger RNA (mRNA) is the intermediary molecule used to carry out this function. mRNA is transcribed from DNA inside the cell nucleus, and contains the same genetic information. It is translocated into the cytoplasm of the cell, where it is used to synthesize the encoded protein.

The human genome is a large and extraordinarily complex library written in DNA. Chromosomal DNA is confined to the nucleus of the cell. The cell nucleus is about 10 microns in diameter (much narrower than the width of a human hair), and amazingly has about 6 meters (almost 20 feet) of double-helix DNA packed inside of it, organized in chromosomes. Humans have 23 pairs of chromosomes, with two copies of each, one of which originated from the father, the other from the mother. (Men are an exception; they have only one copy of the Y chromosome, and a single X chromosome.) Human chromosome 2 contains DNA encoding the lactase protein.

Human genes are generally subject to extremely complicated controls on their expression. "Expression" usually means that a protein, such as an enzyme, is translated from a sequence of codons in the gene. Without very strict control of gene expression, cells would grow and behave chaotically, and complex organisms could not exist. A breakdown in this control of gene expression is characteristic of cancer. These complex genetic control systems are responsible for a single fertilized egg (initially a single cell) developing into an incredibly complex newborn with trillions of cells, and they allow cells in adults to remain dedicated to specific functions, such as fighting infections or producing digestive enzymes. These genetic controls are encoded in specific regulatory regions of DNA. These are areas of DNA that do not encode specific proteins, but serve as switches that turn genes on or off. Frequently control of genes is exerted by proteins that recognize these stretches of regulatory DNA, and bind to specific sequences of nucleotides in the DNA. Depending on the specific control mechanism, such binding of a protein may cause a gene to be expressed more actively, or it may repress expression of the gene. A single gene may be controlled by numerous regions of regulatory DNA, some upregulating gene expression and others downregulating it. The cumulative and sometimes opposing effects of these regulatory regions determines the overall activity level of the gene. It is worth noting that DNA binding regions are just one tool for controlling gene expression; other mechanisms include coating the DNA with inactivating proteins, attaching methyl groups to specific DNA bases, controlling the translation of messenger RNA, production of interfering RNA's, and regulating the functions of proteins produced from the messenger RNA. Overall control of gene expression is an area of continuing scientific discovery, and far too complex to be given justice here.

All humans have lactase genes with roughly the same DNA sequence. Like most human genes, lactase is controlled by a complex regulatory system. The normal result of this regulatory system is that, although the gene is present in every cell in the body, lactase is produced only in certain cells in the tips of the villi, the finger-like projections that line the small intestine. Furthermore the production of lactase in this small area of tissue generally occurs only during infancy and early childhood. As noted previously the DNA regions responsible for controlling lactase production are located in same region of chromosome 2 that carries the lactase gene, but some of the control regions are located a considerable distance from the gene itself (about 14,000 base pairs, or enough DNA in theory to encode several proteins). The following sections will explore the specific DNA mutations that result in lactase persisting into adulthood, and current thinking about how these mutations cause this change.

THE SEARCH FOR THE CAUSE OF ADULT LACTASE PERSISTENCE

The current understanding of the physiology of lactose tolerance and intolerance matured in the 1960's, although scientists in the early 1900's described the presence or absence of lactase in the intestines of juvenile and mature animals.[51] By the 1960's scientists had determined that the lactase persistence trait was genetically transmitted and inherited in a simple dominant manner. Only one copy of a chromosome carrying the then unknown sequence for lactase persistence had to be inherited from a parent in order for a child to be lactase persistent. Identification of this dominant trait triggered a long quest to understand the genetics of lactase persistence. In 1966, Drs. Theodore Bayless and Norman Rosensweig at Johns Hopkins University hypothesized that persistence was under genetic control, based on the strong differences that they saw among ethnic groups.[52] Subsequent work showed that the lactase obtained from intestinal biopsies of persistent individuals was biochemically indistinguishable from the very low levels of lactase isolated from non-persistent individuals.[53] This suggested that the difference was not in the enzyme itself. In 1981, Dr. John Johnson of the University of New Mexico speculated that lactase persistence arose from a mutation in a regulatory gene that controlled lactase synthesis.[54] A quest to identify the causative mutation began in the early 1980's, but this riddle remained unresolved for another 20 years. Progress in this area was initially slow because of the limitations of the molecular biology tools then available. The pace of research quickened markedly as more sophisticated tools for DNA cloning and sequencing became available. However, sequencing of the DNA of the lactase gene and the immediately surrounding areas still did not identify any changes that corresponded to lactase persistence or non-persistence.[55] Dr. Edward Hollox and colleagues sequenced this region in DNA samples from 1338 subjects. In 2001 they reported that in Europeans lactase persistence was linked to inheritance of a region of DNA containing 70,000 base pairs that surrounded the lactase gene.[56] This indicated that the genetic change for persistence was located somewhere in this region. However, they found many variations in DNA sequences in this area, and they lacked a way to find the specific, causative DNA change.

This puzzle was finally solved in 2002 in a massive and elegant experiment conducted by an international group of scientists led by the late Dr. Leena Peltonen at the University of Helsinki.[57] They identified nine Finnish families that contained mixtures of lactase persistent and non-persistent individuals, and in about 125 of these family members they sequenced 47,000 base pair sections of DNA that contained the lactase gene and surrounding areas. They were able to track both lactase status and DNA sequences across multiple generations. They discovered over 50 DNA variations in this region among their pool of subjects. However, analysis of the huge dataset revealed that a mutation in a single DNA base in an area remote from the lactase gene was invariably associated with lactase persistence in these Finnish families. They expanded this investigation to include Italians and African Americans. In these new groups, lactase persistence was associated with the same mutation originally detected in the lactase persistent Finnish family members. Individuals who lacked this mutation were invariably lactase non-persistent. The DNA change responsible for lactase persistence in most Europeans was now known, but another decade would pass before emergence of a clear understanding of how this DNA mutation caused lactase persistence.

At this time geneticists knew that some African populations, particularly in East Africa, contained lactase persistent individuals and in these populations the DNA sequences of the area around the lactase gene were vastly different from the Finnish population. They quickly realized that this single mutation first found in Finns did not occur in most of these lactase-persistent Africans. These populations were later found to have several distinct mutations that produced lactase persistence, leading to a much more complicated story. However, the Peltonen publication was a milestone in human genetics, and this identification of a specific mutation conferring adult lactase persistence led to a huge expansion of research in this area.

GENETICS OF LACTASE PERSISTENCE

The various mutations conferring adult lactase persistence result from changes in single DNA base pairs, the smallest alteration possible in the genetic language. All of these mutations involve one of the four nucleotide bases (adenine, thymine, cytosine, and guanine) being replaced by another one of these four. Such DNA alterations are described as single nucleotide polymorphisms, or "SNP's" (pronounced "snips"). SNP's are alleles, or variations, of genes, and they are very common in the human genome. Complete DNA sequencing of the 46 chromosomes of a fairly small group (270 individuals) of geographically diverse humans revealed about 7,000,000 unique SNP's in this group. The total number of SNP's scattered through the world's peoples is far greater.[58] To date, scientists have discovered five separate SNP mutations that result in adult lactase persistence.

These five SNP's are all located in a tiny stretch of DNA covering 101 bases in a regulatory region about 14,000 bases upstream from the beginning of the lactase gene. The convention for naming these SNP's is a combination of the distance (in nucleotide bases) from the beginning of the lactase gene, and a letter code for the nucleotide change involved in the SNP. For example, the most common mutation for lactase persistence is the SNP -13,910 T. The minus sign means that the SNP is located 13,910 bases before (or upstream from) the start of the lactase gene (DNA is generally read in a specific direction, and sites upstream from the lactase gene are indicated by minus ("-")). "T" is an abbreviation for thymidine, one of the four DNA bases mentioned previously. The human genome before the appearance of lactase persistence contained a cytosine base at position -13,910. Individuals who have the original -13,910 C genotype are lactase non-persistent (unless they carry one of the other four known persistence SNP's as detailed later). In summary, the simple change from a cytosine to a thymidine base at this position renders an individual lactase persistent. Someone with the genotype -13,910 T on a least one copy of chromosome 2 produces abundant lactase in adulthood, whereas the adult who has the -13,910 C genotype on both copies of chromosome 2 lacks functional levels of intestinal lactase.

The roughly 14,000 DNA base pairs that separate the -13,910 T SNP from the beginning of the lactase gene carry out other functions. Oddly, the 101 base pair region containing all of the lactase persistence SNP's is located inside a gene with a far different function. Eukaryotic genes typically consist of lengths of DNA that encode portions of proteins (these DNA segments are known as "exons") that are interspersed with segments of DNA known as "introns" that do not code for the protein. A single gene may contain large numbers of introns and exons. When messenger RNA is transcribed from a gene, all this DNA, both exons and introns, is copied into the messenger RNA. Then, highly specific enzymes (nucleases) splice out the introns, and string the exons together into the messenger RNA strand that is actually used to synthesize the gene's encoded protein. All of the known lactase persistence SNP's are located within the thirteenth intron of the gene for a protein known as Minichromosome Maintenance Protein 6 (MCM-6). MCM-6 is one of a large group of proteins involved in the copying of DNA during cell division. Again, this gene is totally unrelated to lactase, and there is no apparent reason why the DNA region that controls the production of lactase should be found within an intron of a totally different protein. This presence of the DNA that controls lactase inside another gene is an illustrative example of how the molecular genetics of humans is extremely complicated, bizarre, and often organizationally awkward. Rather than being the product of "intelligent design," the human genome appears to be a vast collection of modifications and reuses of existing DNA that have resulted from billions of years of natural selection acting on mutations and DNA rearrangements. Human evolution is basically a random process in which some of these accidentally occurring DNA changes provide a selective benefit to an individual in a particular environment (such as the constant presence of fresh milk).

HOW A SNP CAUSES LACTASE PERSISTENCE

This DNA in the thirteenth intron of MCM serves as binding sites for multiple control proteins (known as promoters, since they promote activity of a gene) that somehow turn on the function of the distant lactase gene. The lactase gene is inactive if the promoter is not attached to this binding site; binding of the promoter serves as an "on" switch for lactase production. DNA is not a stiff rod, but rather an extremely flexible fiber that can twist around on itself (this is obvious from the six meters of DNA jammed into every tiny nucleus). Perhaps inside the cells of the intestinal villi, this MCM-6 intron actually ends up in close proximity to the lactase gene, somehow orchestrating control of its expression.

The expression of DNA and production of proteins is controlled by many processes aside from the control proteins just noted. Another regulatory process is the attachment of methyl groups (CH_3) to specific bases in the DNA chain. These methylations are part of a phenomenon known as "epigenetics," which are changes that can affect long-term activity of genes, even though no change in the DNA sequences are involved. Some methylations are copied each time that the chromosome is duplicated during cell division. In this manner methylation-produced changes in gene activity may persist over the lifetime of an organism, or even be transferred to succeeding generations. The environment experienced by a parent, or perhaps a grandparent, can change the methylation of their DNA, and these changes may be passed on to the children or grandchildren. This is a mechanism for adapting to short-term environmental changes or temporarily altering the function of a gene. Methylation contrasts strongly with natural selection based on changes in DNA sequences, which are permanent and typically take many generations to become widespread.[59] Also, the pattern of methylation in an organism's DNA appears to change inexorably with age (epigenetic aging), and may contribute to the unavoidable declines of aging.

Recent research by a consortium of researchers in Canada and Lithuania demonstrated that methylation patterns in the thirteenth MCM intron, home of all the lactase persistence SNP's, are influenced by the presence of one of these SNP's.[60] Their work suggests that as children grow through the usual age of weaning and enter into childhood, there is a gradual increase in the amount of methylation in this region of DNA. The accumulating methylation makes binding of promoters for the lactase gene more and more difficult. This results in less and less expression of the gene, and hence less intestinal lactase, as methylation builds up with increasing age.

These researchers developed two lines of evidence to support this theory. First, they collected cells from the jejunum (the section of the small intestine that produces lactase) of infant (6 day old) and adult (60 day old) mice and examined the methylation pattern in this intron of MCM-6. The adult mice (which are of course lactase non-producers) had far higher levels of methylation in this control region than did the infant mice. The organization of this area of chromosome 2 is very similar in most mammals, so these results are relevant to humans. The second line of evidence is human data. They analyzed intestinal biopsies collected from adult Lithuanian patients undergoing weight reduction surgery, and examined the extent of methylation in this intron. The investigators also sequenced patient DNA samples to identify the individuals that possessed the - 13,910 T SNP for adult lactase persistence. Compared to patients who were not lactase persistent, those with the persistence SNP had far lower levels of DNA methylation in this region. The authors did not have access to jejunal biopsy samples from young children, but likely these would show the same low levels of methylation observed in infant mice. Thus the ultimate cause of lactase non-persistence, and any ensuing lactose intolerance, appears to be the accumulation of methyl groups in a small area of DNA.

Other research has provided insight into why adults with the -13,910 T SNP have decreased methylation in this area. A group of researchers in Denmark and the United Kingdom determined that this SNP increases the strength of binding of promoter proteins to this control region in the thirteenth MCM intron.[61] This tighter binding blocks access to DNA by the methylating enzymes. This firm binding of specific promoter proteins is the mechanism that limits methylation. In summary, stronger promoter binding caused by the SNP limits the accumulation of methyl groups that cause children to stop producing lactase, thus allowing production of lactase to continue in adulthood.

The slow accumulation of methylation in this intron in lactose non-absorbers may account for why the transition from a lactose tolerant toddler to a lactose intolerant schoolchild is often a gradual process, with the condition sometimes developing over years. In addition, different populations may differ in the age of onset of intestinal lactase deficiency, and in the rapidity of the conversion to non-digesting status (although data supporting these hypotheses are limited). If true, this may reflect differing rates of methylation in these populations, possibly reflecting differences in genes, nutrition, or other lifestyle factors. There is clearly more to learn about this story. Hopefully, in the future researchers will explore the timing of lactase shutdown in various non-persistent populations and develop a mechanistic understanding of any variability.

The preceding discussion summarizes what is currently known about the genetic causes of adult lactase persistence or non-persistence, and admittedly simplifies the story. Other control mechanisms for the lactase gene are known, and potentially these could also play a role in lactase persistence, or the amount of expression of lactase. Like most processes in biology, this one is probably much more complex than we realize, and it is certain that this story will become even more elaborate in the future.

ONE COPY OF A SNP, OR TWO? DOES IT MATTER?

Humans, like all vertebrate animals, are diploid; that is, they have two copies of every chromosome and thus two copies of every DNA sequence (again, an exception is male mammals, which have a single "X" chromosome, and a single largely non-functional "Y" chromosome). Since humans have two copies of chromosome 2 containing the lactase gene, they obviously carry two copies of the lactase gene and the surrounding DNA. The DNA position at -13,910 may contain cytosine (C) or thymidine (T). Therefore three different combinations are possible: C+C, C+T, or T+T (these are more conveniently expressed as C/C, C/T, or T/T). The -13,910 T SNP is genetically dominant, and an individual who is either C/T or T/T is lactase persistent.

A logical question is whether there is a difference in lactose metabolism between individuals who have T/T genetic makeup at -13,910 and those with the C/T genotype (only one copy carries the persistence SNP). To answer this question, researchers in Sweden collected medical records from a large number of patients previously tested for lactose malabsorption by a lactose challenge test. As detailed later, this is a physiological test for evaluating lactose metabolism,[62] and increasing breath hydrogen levels reflect decreased amounts of intestinal lactase. They also sequenced DNA from consenting individuals in this group to determine if they were C/C, C/T, or T/T for the -13,910 SNP, and compared breath hydrogen levels and symptoms observed in the lactose challenge test for the three groups. Individuals who were T/T had the lowest breath hydrogen levels after lactose consumption, indicating a high level of lactose digestion. C/T individuals had slightly higher breath hydrogen levels, but the C/C group had hydrogen levels about ten times that of the T/T group. There was no observed difference in patient-reported symptom severity between the C/T and T/T groups, though this is a subjective, notoriously inaccurate measure. Thus individuals with only one copy of the lactase persistence SNP have lower levels of intestinal lactase in comparison to those who carried two copies, and potentially these individuals could be more sensitive to dairy digestion problems under some conditions such as secondary lactose intolerance.

DIVERSITY OF LACTASE PERSISTENCE

Currently five SNP's, all within this very short length of DNA, are known to confer adult lactase persistence. This proves that lactase persistence has evolved independently at least five times. Also, based on the geographic distribution of populations containing lactase persistent individuals, it is possible that some of these five mutations appeared multiple times in different populations, so there may have been more than five independent origins. The fact that two individuals possess the same SNP does not necessarily mean that they inherited it from some remote common ancestor.

The widespread emergence of adult lactase persistence was the result of ongoing human evolution in Europe, Africa, and Asia in response to the domestication of dairy animals such as cattle, sheep, goats, and camels. The geographic dispersal of the respective SNP's accompanied the spread of domesticated animals that could serve as a source of milk. The next two chapters trace the histories of these multiple origins of lactase persistence. The development of lactase persistence in Europe will be considered first since this area has benefited from the most research. This order of presentation is not because of cultural bias, but rather because this story of the causative SNP is simplest, best understood, and provides a perspective for the other SNP's.

5 Emergence of Lactase Persistence in Europe

LACTASE PERSISTENCE FIRST APPEARED IN CENTRAL EUROPE

The appearance of lactase persistence closely followed the domestication and spread of cattle and other ruminants. Domestication of cattle occurred about 10,300-10,800 years ago in the Fertile Crescent.[63] Lactase persistence appeared in cattle-rearing populations a few thousand years later; perhaps during this time human selection of these newly domesticated animals resulted in animals sufficiently docile for milking. Dr. Yuval Itan, a geneticist at University College in London, and colleagues used data on the distribution of the -13,910 C/T alleles in modern populations and the history of the development of agriculture to develop a computer model to predict the time and location of the first appearance of lactase persistence in European populations.[64] Their simulations indicated that this SNP appeared between 6200 and 8600 years before the present, with the most probable location of its origin somewhere in the central Balkans and central Europe (encompassing the southern portions of present day Germany and Poland). As noted in the previous chapter, agriculture and domesticated cattle reached this part of Europe about 8500 years ago, so lactase persistence appeared soon after dairy animals became established there. Thus according to this work the -13,910 T SNP appears to have originated in Europe, and not the Fertile Crescent where cattle were first domesticated several thousand years earlier.

Sequencing of DNA extracted from human bones recovered from archeological excavations in Central and Eastern Europe provides confirmation of this timing.[65] Archeological or radiocarbon (^{14}C) data were used to date eight human bones from three different sites as being between 7000 and 8000 years old, about the time that domesticated large animals and agriculture reached Europe. DNA extracted from these bones was sequenced. All eight were -13,910 C, indicating that the individuals were not lactase persistent. Although this is a limited data set, it indicates that lactase persistence was not widespread in Europe before the introduction of pastoralism and agriculture. What cannot be determined is whether the -13,910 T SNP appeared almost simultaneously with the origin of dairy culture, or whether this SNP was lurking at a low level in this population, awaiting a selective advantage that caused it to become more predominant in populations over time.

The lack of widespread distribution of the -13,910 T SNP before ruminant animal domestication argues that dairying drove the spread of this SNP, rather than the pre-existing existence of this SNP in certain populations facilitating the spread of dairying and milk consumption. The earlier scientific literature had featured a debate of this "directionality" issue, but sequencing ancient DNA has resolved this.[66]

In central Europe the recently arrived agriculturists were beginning to use milk as a food source. Somewhere in this population, very rare individuals, perhaps just one, carried the -13,910T SNP that conferred lactase persistence. Within an extremely short period (in an evolutionary sense), the descendants of these lactase-persistent pioneers increased in number dramatically, to the point that some contemporary European populations are almost all lactase persistent. It is widely recognized that lactase persistence spread more rapidly than any other known recent human genetic change.[67] This SNP must have provided extremely powerful selective advantages in the agricultural or pastoral populations where it appeared. Just what these selective advantages were is not at all clear. The ability to utilize the full nutritional benefits of dairy, particularly fresh milk, could have driven this natural selection.

Genetic analysis has highlighted the strength of the selective advantage for persistence. Geneticists utilize a tool known as haplotype analysis for measuring how quickly a genetic change proliferates in a population. Haplotypes are sections of DNA that are passed down intact through generations largely without being recombined during the meiosis involved in the production of eggs and sperm.

Meiosis is a process in which haploid (that is, having a single set of chromosomes) sperm and eggs are produced from the normally diploid (two sets of chromosomes) cells of the parents. During meiosis, the matching chromosomes of each pair tightly align, and recombination occurs across the paired DNA strands to cut and paste matching segments of DNA between the chromosomes. Genetic information is swapped back and forth between these paired chromosomes in a very orderly manner. As a result meiosis produces chromosomes that are mosaics of DNA regions that came from both of the individual's parents. After meiosis, the unpaired recombined chromosome is incorporated into a forming egg or sperm. Fertilization of the egg by the sperm restores the normal diploid status.

Although haplotypes are regions of DNA that are typically passed through generations without being altered by recombination during meiosis, recombination within haplotypes does occur occasionally. Since recombination occurs during each round of meiosis that creates the egg and sperm for each new generation, the DNA diversity of the haplotype increases over time because of these occasional recombinations within the haplotype. If a mutation (such as adult lactase persistence) is present within a long uniform haplotype, this is an indication that the mutation is fairly recent. Also, the widespread presence of the same intact haplotype in a population indicates a strong genetic selective advantage. The haplotype containing the lactase persistence mutation must have conferred a very powerful selective advantage in these pastoral Europeans, because very few recombination events accumulated within it.

Drawing on data from many hundreds of people from diverse populations, geneticists at Harvard University examined DNA sequences for a large section of human chromosome 2 containing the lactase gene.[68] They found that the -13,910 T SNP was contained in a very large haplotype containing over 800,000 DNA base pairs. They further analyzed the genetic data with a set of complex mathematical and statistical tests (these are the toolbox of the modern geneticists) to determine a Coefficient of Selection (CoS) for this mutation. The CoS is a measure of the evolutionary selective advantage of a DNA change (such as a SNP). The greater the selective advantage in the tested population, the higher the CoS will be. The CoS for the lactase persistence SNP was between 0.14 and 0.15 for a pooled European population, and between 0.09 and 0.19 for a Scandinavian population, indicating a strong selective advantage. The Harvard scientists concluded that lactase persistence "represents one of the strongest signals of recent positive selection yet documented in the genome" (p.1118). A compelling comparison would be genetic resistance to malaria. Malaria is a significant cause of human mortality, and two genetic mutations that provide some resistance to malaria are known: glucose-6 phosphate deficiency (G6PD) deficiency, and the sickle cell trait. The coefficient of selection of G6PD is estimated at 0.02-0.05, and 0.05-0.18 for sickle cell. Therefore, in these northern European populations, adult lactase persistence provided a greater selective advantage than that provided in other populations by some resistance to malaria, a frequently fatal disease. However, it must be noted that lactase persistence does not have any known deleterious effects, whereas the sickle cell trait causes severe anemia that may be fatal in homozygotes.

WHAT DROVE THE RAPID SPREAD OF LACTASE PERSISTENCE IN NORTHERN EUROPE?

Although lactase persistence spread amazingly rapidly (from an evolutionary perspective) through some early Northern European pastoral populations, we can only speculate on the selective advantage that drove this. Quite possibly multiple advantages acted in concert. The following paragraphs present several hypotheses to account for this spread. All of these are largely speculative, and the real reason or reasons may be unknowable.

European archeological evidence indicates that the spread of dairying (particularly cattle) closely accompanied the spread of agriculture. This early agriculture was based on a few principal crops (wheat, barley, peas, and lentils), and could have been protein and nutrient poor, in comparison to a hunter-gatherer diet rich in animal protein. For these farmers, the ability of the lactase persistent individuals to utilize more effectively the protein and nutrient content of fresh dairy may have provided a selective advantage. A related possibility is that this agricultural diet was low in calcium, and consuming the calcium in fresh milk could have conferred a health benefit.

Another hypothesis relates to diseases spread through drinking water. Settled agriculture, and increased population densities, may have resulted in pollution of water sources, and water-borne infections could have caused high mortality in poorly nourished people living under crowded conditions, as is the case today in many impoverished societies. Consumption of fresh milk would partially replace drinking of contaminated water, providing a selective advantage to the milk drinker.

Yet another hypothesis is that the vitamin D content of milk was of particular benefit to populations inhabiting the higher latitudes of Europe where wintertime sunshine is scarce, and the ability to produce vitamin D in the skin in limited.[69] The levels of vitamin D naturally found in milk could have been protective against deficiencies. However, the vitamin D content of milk is quite low (readers in the United States and Canada may consider milk to be a good source of vitamin D, but this is due to artificial fortification). Meat has a higher vitamin D content than milk, and eggs and seafood are also very high compared to milk. The fact that lactase persistence also spread in parts of tropical Africa, where abundant sunshine should lead to adequate vitamin D levels, also contradicts this hypothesis.

Increased total caloric intake may have provided a benefit to adults with lactase persistence. An individual who is lactase persistent can obtain the full caloric benefit of the lactose and other nutrients in fresh milk. In contrast, these lactose calories are largely lost in a non-persistent individual. Although the body may scavenge some calories from the products of lactose fermentation in the colon, even this may be difficult if dairy consumption induces diarrhea. In addition, diarrhea associated with lactose intolerance, accompanied by more rapid passage of ingested material through the small intestine, may have decreased the digestion of the protein and fat in milk. Somewhat detracting from this hypothesis are reports that people who are lactose malabsorbers are able to consume moderate quantities of milk, without adverse effects particularly if consumed with other foods.[70]

A supply of milk from dairy animals may have increased the fecundity of women, certainly a huge reproductive advantage. As noted in the first chapter, nursing causes hormonal changes that prevent ovulation, and a nursing mother does not generally become pregnant. The presence of milk from domestic animals may have allowed the mother to transition infants to this milk supply at an early age. This earlier weaning would result in the woman ovulating again, and becoming pregnant. This effect would have tended to increase the population of dairying societies, and may have helped account for their rapid spread. Perhaps lactase persistence in infants and toddlers contributed to this benefit by keeping them free of lactose intolerance symptoms while consuming dairy during the period of weaning. Although persistence does not supply a direct selective advantage here, the increased presence of milk in a population of lactose persistent adults may have led to more cow's milk consumption by infants and toddlers, allowing them to wean from their mothers earlier.

Natural selection in these early agricultural societies may have acted most strongly on children. Infant and childhood mortality rates are high today in less developed societies, and similar mortality may have existed among these early farmers. Dr. Steven Pray at Southwestern Oklahoma State University proposed a hypothesis of increased survival of lactase persistent children during famine.[71] Children in early pastoral societies before the expansion of the lactase SNP would have lost lactase at about the time of weaning. During a famine (assuming that cows still produced milk), that child could consume milk, but would likely to develop diarrhea from the lactose, and regardless could not benefit from the substantial calories provided by the lactose in milk. However, the child with the mutation for lactase persistence could receive the full nutritional benefit of milk. Famine could have been very common in these early agricultural societies, particularly in more northern or drought-prone areas with uncertain growing conditions. A reliance on only a handful of food crops would have made these groups highly vulnerable to crop losses resulting from weather, insects, or diseases. Abundant archeological evidence indicates that warfare and accompanying massacres were disturbingly common among these Neolithic societies, and such calamities could have been highly disruptive to food production.[72] Under such conditions of frequent famine and conflict, these lactase persistent children would have had a powerful advantage, and survived to pass this trait on to their own children.

Another possible source of natural selection for lactase persistence is a protective effect against birth defects in children of milk-drinking mothers. This leads to an admittedly complex hypothesis. Researchers participating in the National Birth Defects Prevention Study (United States) examined the frequency of neural tube defects (NTD) in the children of non-Hispanic white women who carried or lacked the -13,910 T SNP for lactase persistence.[73] NTD occur during the first month of pregnancy, and deficiency in folate (vitamin B-9) is a major cause. NTD result in a number of debilitating conditions, including spina bifida.

Investigators found that NTD were more common in the offspring of women who were not lactase persistent. Importantly, NTD incidence was increased only in the offspring of lactase non-persistent women who consumed 12 or more grams of lactose per day (equivalent to a cup of milk). In non-persistent women who consumed less lactose, the frequency of NTD was similar to that of lactase persistent women. The authors speculated that lactose consumption by pregnant women could cause gastrointestinal changes that interfere with absorption of nutrients such as folate, increasing NTD risk. Notably, the researchers also evaluated a group of US women with Hispanic backgrounds. In these women, the absence of lactase persistence was not associated with increased NTD risk, and in fact it seemed to have a slight protective effect. The authors proposed that dietary differences or socioeconomic stratification could be involved in the discrepant results between these two groups.

As with all findings based on a single study, these NTD results must be interpreted with caution. However, they do suggest an interesting rationale about how diets of the early European dairy consumers could have produced a natural selection for the -13,910 T SNP. In these groups, milk was routinely available, and many people may have consumed substantial amounts despite being lactose malabsorbers. Perhaps they did not develop symptoms, or possibly accepted these symptoms as a trade-off to suffering hunger or protein deprivation. The higher incidence of birth defects in non-persistent women consuming considerable amounts of lactose led to poorer survival of their offspring, compared to lactase persistent women, providing a natural selection for the persistence SNP.

Although the reasons for the astonishingly rapid spread of lactase persistence in some early pastoral societies remain unknown, persistence provided the basis for a culture of dairying that profoundly affected the structures of these societies, and even the landscape. Regardless of the specific selective advantages, this is an insightful story of how human cultural evolution (the domestication of ruminants) led to a genetic change in humans.

THE -13,910 T SNP RAPIDLY SPREAD IN EUROPE

The -13,910 T SNP dispersed broadly from its putative origin in central Europe, with an incidence in contemporary populations that varies widely. As shown in Table 1 on page 67, the highest penetration is in northwest Europe, with about 95% of the Irish population being lactase persistent. Penetration is lower in southern Europe. As noted in the previous chapter, farming and ruminant domestication appear to have spread into Europe from the Fertile Crescent by two routes: up the Danube Valley, and along the shores of the Mediterranean. Populations derived from this Danube route generally carry higher levels of lactase persistence. This may be due to greater selective advantage for persistence in their ancestors, or possibly from what geneticists describe as the founder effect: the genes present in the first inhabitants of an area become predominant in the later, greatly expanded population.[74] The population at the leading edge of the Danube route may have had a high penetration of this SNP, and it became similarly common in their descendants who expanded into northern and northeastern Europe. Today this SNP is less common in the European countries bordering the Mediterranean. Lactase persistence appears to have first appeared in central Europe, and the original agricultural settlers in the Mediterranean may have had little genetic exchange with this population. In addition, cattle rearing for dairy production appears to have been less important in the Mediterranean. Although cattle were the economically predominant domesticated animal in northern Europe, sheep and goats were more common in the Mediterranean. Although these animals produce milk, the smaller volumes may have deceased the impact on human nutrition. Perhaps the drier climate of this region may have limited the forage available for cattle. In Roman Italy, cheese was made mainly from sheep and goat milk. Romans raised cattle mainly as draft animals, though some milk was produced. Perhaps the lower significance of dairy in the Mediterranean diet decreased the selective advantage of the -13,910 T SNP. Also, other environmental factors such as less frequent conditions that produced famines may have decreased the selective advantage in comparison to northern Europe.

Table 1: Frequency of -13,910 T SNP in Some European Populations	
Location	Frequency (%)*
Ireland	95
Scandinavia	82
Southern Britain	73
Orkney Islands	69
French Basque	67
Germany	56
France	43
Northern Italy	36
Greece	13
Sardinia	7
Tuscany	6
Turkey	3
Adapted from Itan, Y, Powell, A, Beaumont, MA, Burger, J, et al. The origins of lactase persistence in Europe, PLoS Computational Biology 5:e1000491 (2009).	
*Percent of population carrying at least one copy of this SNP.	

EUROPEAN PASTORALISTS STROVE TO INCREASE MILK PRODUCTION

The high frequency of lactase persistence in northern Europe and the economic benefits of dairy products may have encouraged farmers to breed cattle that were better milk producers, leaving a genetic imprint that remains in the dairy breeds raised there today. Generally, cattle native to northern Europe have decreased overall genetic diversity, in comparison to the original site of domestication in the Fertile Crescent. This is to be expected, since the animals that were used to establish the first European populations were only a small subgroup of the original domesticated population. However, diversity in the genes related to milk production is actually higher in cattle breeds developed in Northern Europe. This likely reflects humans selecting breeding cows from their best milk producers, measured in terms of either total amount, or length of time of production after calving. Humans may have selected cows with rare variants or mutations that enhanced milk production. The overall result of these selection efforts was an overall increase specifically in the diversity of genes related to milk production.[75]

These Northern Europeans also used husbandry practices to increase milk production. When cattle are weaned, this dietary change is recorded in proteins of the dentin of the growing teeth. Nitrogen is a key component of proteins, and exists primarily in nature as the ^{14}N isotope, though a small amount of ^{15}N is also present. Both isotopes are present in the proteins produced by plants. When animals eat this plant matter, amino acids containing ^{15}N are selectively incorporated into animal protein. Consequently, the protein in cow's milk is higher in the ratio of ^{15}N to ^{14}N than is the forage on which the cow grazed. Calves gradually incorporate proteins (mostly collagen) into the growing dentin in their teeth. An analysis of the ^{15}N/^{14}N ratio of the dentin in different portions of the growing tooth indicates the approximate age of the animal at the time of weaning, when they no longer consume relatively ^{15}N-rich milk. French researchers analyzed the ^{15}N/^{14}N ratio of the second molar of cattle teeth excavated from a 6000-year-old settlement near Paris. The second molar is ideal for this analysis, since it develops gradually between two months and two years of age. Compared to modern cattle, this ratio indicated that these dairymen weaned calves at an earlier age than is typical for modern cattle. This suggests that in this agricultural settlement, farmers used early weaning to reserve milk production for human consumption.[76]

LACTASE PERSISTENCE IN EUROPE MAY HAVE TRIGGERED GENETIC CHANGES IN IRON ABSORPTION

The appearance of lactase persistence and the accompanying increased dairy consumption may have triggered additional genetic changes in the affected populations. One of these is an alteration in iron metabolism. People who trace their ancestry to the British Isles or Scandinavia, in comparison to the rest of the world's population, have a much higher incidence of hemochromatosis, a disease caused by the excessive accumulation of iron in the body. In a strange twist to the story of the spread of lactase persistence in Europe, hemochromatosis may be a side effect of another genetic change that helped early agriculturalists in northern Europe to adapt to a high dairy diet.[77] As discussed in the previous chapter, the Paleolithic diet was high in meat. In comparison, the northern European Neolithic diet was high in grains (especially wheat) and dairy products, and much lower in meat. Meat and some seafoods are a rich source of iron. In contrast, grains contain little iron. Furthermore, the surface of grain kernels contains phytates, which are substances that bind to, and prevent absorption of, several minerals including iron. Dairy products from cattle are low in iron but high in calcium. The proportion of iron absorbed from human milk is about two and a half times higher than the portion absorbed from cow's milk. The low bioavailability of iron in cow's milk appears to result from the high level of calcium interfering with its absorption.[78] These populations that had adopted a diet of grain and dairy may have suffered widespread iron deficiency, and children weaned onto cow's milk at an early stage were especially vulnerable to iron deficiency. This anemia causes fatigue, lethargy, and poor concentration in both children and adults. Babies born to anemic mothers tend to be underweight and more prone to health problems.

Conclusive diagnosis of anemia from ancient skeletal remains is problematic. Iron tends to leach from bones very readily, so determining the iron content of skeletons is not useful. However, chronic iron anemia is associated with two abnormalities of the bones of the skull, porotic hyperostosis and criba orbitalia. The usual basis for diagnosing anemia from skeletal remains is the presence of spongy areas in the interior of these bones. However, this approach is controversial, as other conditions may cause these skeletal anomalies.[79] This is perhaps the weakest point in the hypothesis associating anemia with a grain-dairy diet in Neolithic groups.

Genetic changes in these northwestern European populations provided a remedy for this possible iron deficiency, although imperfect (as is often the case with evolution's solutions). A gene on human chromosome 6 known as HFE is involved in absorption of dietary iron. This gene produces a protein that regulates the activity of transferrin, another protein that carries iron through the circulatory system. The regulation of iron absorption is complex, and normally the HFE protein provides a safeguard to prevent the absorption of too much iron. In Europe, two different mutations (the C282Y and H63D alleles) appeared in the

HFE gene, and both had the effect of increasing iron absorption. C282Y appears to have originated in the last 3000 – 5000 years in northeastern Europe, and in some of these populations it is now present in about 10% of individuals. In contrast, H63D is older and more widely distributed in European populations, but never achieves the level of population penetrance of C282Y. Both alleles confer improved iron status on individuals consuming a low iron diet. Just as in the case of lactase persistence, the appearance of random DNA changes and subsequent selective pressures acting on them provided a solution to a nutritional problem, this time an iron deficiency caused by a diet reliant on grains and dairy.

In the grain and dairy rich diets of the Neolithic British Isles and Scandinavia, carriers of these mutations of HFE were able to absorb more of the meager amounts of iron in their diets, and they were more resistant to the fatigue and other afflictions related to anemia in these societies. Selective pressure for these mutations obviously appeared more recently than selection for lactase persistence. Perhaps this is a reason that these iron absorption mutations have not spread through populations as extensively as lactase persistence. It is unclear if there was just one original C282Y mutation or several, but this trait spread widely in the dairying populations of northern Europe. Statistical analyses of the frequencies of lactase persistence and HFE mutations show a very high correlation for C282Y, indicating a possible natural selection for improved iron absorption in these lactase persistent populations. Cultural changes eventually obviated the selective advantages of these HFE mutations. With onset of the Iron Age, iron cooking ware became widespread in Europe about 2500 years ago, and iron leaching from these utensils helped to correct the dearth of iron in these diets. However, despite the use of iron cookware signs of anemia are found in many European skeletons from the Roman, medieval, and early industrial times. Iron deficiency anemia remains a problem in many developing areas, and also some individuals in the developed world.

Lactase persistence is an overwhelmingly beneficial trait in the modern world. The same cannot be said for the HFE mutations, since these can lead to too much iron absorption from a diet with better iron sources. Individuals who carry a mutation in HFE for increased iron absorption on only one copy of chromosome 6 (heterozygotes) generally suffer no negative consequences. However, in these heterozygotes excess alcohol consumption may trigger a number of maladies related to excess iron accumulation. In contrast, those who carry HFE mutations on both copies of chromosome 6 (homozygotes) may develop hemochromatosis, or iron overload. This is a potentially lethal accumulation of iron in the liver and kidneys. Fortunately, only about 1% of the homozygotes develop clinical symptoms of hemochromatosis; these include fatigue, liver cirrhosis and cancer, and heart disease. Disease incidence in homozygotes appears to be determined by a number of other genetic modifications, as well as lifestyle factors. Symptoms of hemochromatosis do not appear until after age 40 in men, and after menopause in women. Due to this late age of onset, the reproductive success of homozygous carriers is not severely affected. This would have helped this mutation spread through these earlier dairying populations.

These agricultural societies dependent on a diet of grain and dairy were apparently successful, and particularly in the British Isles they quickly replaced the hunter-gatherer tradition. However, this diet had a downside of iron deficiency; the natural selection for increased iron absorption resulting from mutations in the HFE gene provided an interesting genetic solution to this problem. This diet probably caused other health problems as well, providing additional opportunities for natural selection in the human gene pool. Perhaps other stories of adaptive genetic changes await discovery.

Lactase persistence in Europe began perhaps as a in a single mutation, the -13,910 T SNP, that appeared in central Europe and radiated outward to dairying populations in all directions. The appearance of lactase persistence in these populations strongly affected these cultures, and led to more genetics changes. The story of lactase persistence in Africa and Asia is even more complex, as revealed in the next chapter.

6 APPEARANCE AND SPREAD OF LACTASE PERSISTENCE IN AFRICA AND ASIA

MULTIPLE SNP's FOR LACTASE PERSISTENCE

The genetic story of lactase persistence in Africa and southwest Asia is both more multifaceted and less well understood than in Europe. Lactase persistence in these adjoining regions arose from a diversity of SNP's, in contrast to the single SNP responsible for persistence in most of Europe. African lactase persistence may be due to any one of five different SNP's (-13910 T, -13907 G, -13915 G, -14009 G, and -14010 C). Table 2 on the following page summarizes the geographic ranges and highest reported frequencies of these SNP's. In some populations, multiple persistence alleles are extant, and the area of greatest genetic diversity is in northeast Africa, particularly the current nations of South Sudan, Ethiopia, and Kenya.[80] In this region some individuals even carry two of these SNP's, one inherited from the mother, and one from the father. Aside from these five SNP's known to be associated with lactase persistence, numerous other rare SNP's have been reported (at -13,913, -14091, -14,107, and -14,176). Whether these SNP's produce persistence is not currently known, and they may instead reflect the vast genetic diversity in African populations.[81]

Table 2: Lactase Persistence SNP's			
SNP	Estimated Age (Years)	Geographic Area (1)	Maximum Population Incidence (2)
-13,910 T	6200-6800	Europe, Mideast, India, Central Asia, North Africa, Cameroon, Chad	90+%
-14,010 C	6000-7500	Large portions of east Africa, southern Africa	50%
-13,915 G	4000	Kenya, Sudan, Ethiopia, Yemen, Saudi Arabia, India	90%
-13,907 G	Unknown	Kenya, Sudan (very limited)	21%
-14,009 G	Unknown	Ethiopia, Sudan	?
1- Geographic range prior to post-1492 European colonial expansion. 2- Highest level of SNP penetration in any studied population.			

The difference in the diversity of lactase persistence in Europe and Africa is intriguing, and multiple factors (including mere chance) may be involved. The European situation may reflect the -13,910 T SNP arising in a single, early pastoral/agricultural population that became extremely successful, and was able to spread its culture and genes over a large geography. As discussed earlier, the herding and farming culture that moved into Europe from the Fertile Crescent largely displaced the hunter-gatherers that had occupied these lands. If the original lactase persistence SNP had appeared in the people living at the advancing edge of agriculture, the SNP could have expanded rapidly as that population increased in numbers to inhabit the new territory (known in genetics as the "founder effect"). In contrast, the situation in Africa reflects the independent development of lactase persistence in multiple populations, with that persistence arising from genetically different SNP's. In much of northern Africa, cattle herding was well established before the SNP's became widespread in populations, and unlike Europe there does not appear to have been a rapid expansion of a particular dairying population with a lactase persistence SNP. Over time, migration and intermixing spread the various persistence SNP's through multiple African populations, giving rise to the robust distribution of SNP's seen there today.

An additional factor underlying the European and African differences may lie in the respective amounts of genetic diversity in these populations. Modern humans first appeared in Africa about 100,000 years ago. The small groups that migrated away from this ancestral home to populate other portions of the globe carried only a fraction of the total genetic diversity of their African ancestors. The African population retained a considerable pool of genetic diversity, as indicated by modern Africans being more genetically diverse than the world's other populations.[82] This leads to the possibility that multiple SNP's conferring lactase persistence could have been quietly lurking in this complex African genetic diversity. The domestication of dairy animals, and the availability of milk, provided the selective advantage that caused the SNP's to become more predominant in these new dairy consuming populations. In contrast, European and central Asian populations lacked this genetic diversity, and a single SNP arising in one of these populations became the source of virtually all lactase persistence in these regions.

THE -14,010 C PERSISTENCE SNP

Researchers at the Max Planck Institute in Germany researched the origin and spread of this SNP, which is the most prevalent of those in Africa.[83] Using DNA samples obtained from diverse people in northeast Africa, they sequenced a region containing the SNP and the adjacent areas. This SNP-containing section of DNA in MCM intron 13 contains short tandem repeats (STR's), which are sections of non-coding DNA. Non-coding DNA is not translated into proteins, and some of it may have no function at all (often referred to as "junk DNA"). Various STR's are common in the human genome, and they tend to accumulate silent mutations (such as SNPs) as DNA is passed down from generation to generation. Thus the sequence diversity among STR's in specific locations provides an indication of how long ago these DNA regions descended from a common ancestral DNA sequence. This analysis of STR variations provides a measure of the degree of relationship among different populations. Enrico Macholdt and colleagues at Max Planck determined that the -14010 C SNP first appeared somewhere in East Africa (most likely in the region occupied by the current countries of Tanzania and Kenya) about 6000-7500 years ago. The natural selection for this SNP was originally weak, but selection later accelerated. This may reflect the SNP initially lying latent in the population, indicating little or no selective advantage. Later selection accelerated with the continued development of a pastoral lifestyle, in which dairy products became more nutritionally important.

One noteworthy group that carries the -14,010 C SNP at a high frequency are the Maasai. These pastoralists currently live in Kenya and Tanzania, though linguistic analysis indicates an origin in more northern Africa. Until recently, the Maasai relied on their livestock for almost their entire diet, and they probably represent an extreme of adaptation to a pastoral lifestyle. In the past they consumed large amounts of fresh and fermented milk, as well as meat and blood. Plant consumption was minimal, and killing wildlife was a violation of their beliefs. In addition to the strong genetic selection for lactase persistence produced by their diet, other adaptive genetic changes have helped the Maasai to thrive on this high fat, high cholesterol diet. Despite fat making up about 60% of their total caloric intake and dietary cholesterol intakes far in excess of levels recommended in the Western diet, total cholesterol levels in Maasai consuming their traditional diet averaged about 135 mg/dl, compared to averages ranging from 160 mg to 266 mg in a group of countries with high fat, Western diets. Triglyceride levels in the Maasai are also low. Their healthy lipid profiles appear to be due to genetic changes in a number of lipid-modifying enzymes.[84] In addition, their health was likely supported by their high activity levels and generally very thin physiques. Recently, increased population and decreased amounts of grazing land have forced the Maasai into more sedentary and agricultural lifestyles that include much more carbohydrate intake. Unfortunately, they may eventually face the complex of diseases associated with modern life.

The previous chapter discussed the dearth of iron in the grain and dairy based diets of Neolithic northwest Europe, and a similar lack of iron would appear to be a threat to the Maasai. However, the Maasai have a long tradition of consuming blood from cattle, or mixing this blood with milk. The consumption of iron-rich blood may have been a cultural adaptation to a dairy diet low in available iron, and there was not the strong selection of mutations enhancing iron absorption that had occurred in northwest Europe.

About 3000 to 4500 years ago people carrying the -14,010 C SNP migrated to southern Africa. Most likely these people (and their cattle) migrated along a narrow elevated corridor of eastern Africa where the tsetse fly does not thrive. Today this SNP is common in some of the indigenous pastoral populations southernmost Africa, including modern Namibia, Botswana, and South Africa. Other DNA evidence supports this hypothesized migration. Traces of Eurasian DNA were introduced into east African populations beginning several thousand years ago, perhaps reflecting human movements through the calm ocean off eastern Africa. Remnants of this same Eurasian DNA are also found in some Southern African populations where -14010 C is widespread. The frequency of lactase persistence in some groups of the Nama people of Namibia is about 50%, indicating a strong natural selection. The Nama are a Bantu-speaking cattle-herding people; this SNP is less common in neighboring groups who remain hunter-gatherers, such as the San. Swedish geneticists used changes in DNA linkages (these are caused by recombination) to estimate that these migrants carrying the -14,010 C SNP reached southern Africa about 1150-1250 years ago.[85] Cattle remains more than 1600 years old have been discovered in South Africa, so possibly cattle reached the southern portion of Africa somewhat before the arrival of lactase persistence. This genetic analysis also indicates that the DNA of the original migrants has been substantially diluted with DNA of the prior inhabitants of the region. This suggests that a group of lactase-persistent pastoralists from eastern Africa assimilated into a larger pre-existing group, who then adopted cattle raising. This genetic dilution should have had the effect of reducing the frequency of the -14,010 C persistence SNP. However, this SNP is now present at a much higher level than would be expected after this population dilution, indicating a strong recent selective advantage for carriers of this SNP. This is similar to the rapid expansion of the -13,910 SNP in Northern European populations.

-13,915 G: THE CAMEL MILK SNP

For many years the laboratory of Dr. Sarah Tischkoff at the University of Pennsylvania has studied the genetics of African populations, and they have spearheaded research on lactase persistence in this region. A massive study lead-authored by Dr. Alessia Ranciaro in that lab provides detail on the geographic distribution of persistence SNP's in Africa, and their likely routes of spread.[86] This group sequenced sections of DNA from 819 individuals from a broad diversity of populations. This sequencing included the MCM6 gene itself as well as flanking regions of DNA that contained four fast evolving segments. This study underlies the current understanding of the distribution of the various African persistence SNP's.

The Penn researchers found that the SNP -13,915 G occurs in portions of Kenya and the Sudan, and is especially common on the Arabian Peninsula. Estimates from genetic linkage data indicate that this SNP first appeared on the Arabian Peninsula about 4000 years ago. The dromedary camel was domesticated in this area about 6000 years ago, and the availability of camel milk could have provided the initial natural selection for the increased frequency of this SNP.

The camel is an alternative to dairy cattle in some very arid areas, and camels are extensively used for dairy in the Mid-East, northern Africa, and in central Asia. For example, in the dry climate of northern Kenya, on an individual basis camels are able to produce far more milk than dairy cattle. Nomadic groups are very reliant on camel milk, and when moving between areas of pasture they can survive for up a month with camel milk as their only sustenance.[87] Lactating camels allowed to drink water for only one hour each week are still able to produce milk, although this milk is more concentrated in nutrients.[88] It should be recognized that dairying in camel-raising regions is not limited to just camels; goats, sheep, and cows (to some extent) are also milked. The distribution of the - 13,915 SNP overlies much of this area where camels are exploited for dairy. The intense utilization of camel milk in these nomadic populations probably provided a strong selection for lactase persistence, analogous to the development of lactase persistence among the early dairy herders of northern Europe. Even though this SNP only appeared about 4000 years ago, Tischkoff and colleagues found it to be present in frequencies of greater than 60% in some tribes of Arabian Peninsula, which is a breathtaking pace for human evolution. A separate study evaluated lactase persistence among Bedouin tribes in Kuwait.[89] In one group, the Mutran, 90% of adults were lactase persistent. Most of these people carried this -13,915 SNP, but some individuals possessed the -13,907 G SNP, which is discussed below. This nomadic group has a heavy consumption of milk products, providing a strong selective pressure for persistence.

OTHER AFRICAN PERSISTENCE SNP's

Dr. Tischkoff's lab found that another persistence SNP, -13,907 G, is limited to a few populations in Ethiopia, Kenya and Sudan, and not found widely outside of Africa. Linguistic patterns and known human migrations suggest that this SNP first appeared in Ethiopia, and then spread south. Interestingly, a few Kenyan individuals carry both -14010 C and -13907 G (on different copies of chromosome 2, one inherited from each parent).

Another genetic study by British, Ethiopian, and Danish researchers led by Dr. Dallas Swallow evaluated the diversity of lactase persistence in Ethiopia.[90] They utilized students from the University of Addis Ababa, who represented a broad cross section of Ethiopian ethnic groups. These researchers performed lactose hydrogen breath tests on these subjects, and also sequenced DNA isolated from swabs taken from inside the cheeks. Analysis of results from 356 subjects indicated the presence of the three African SNP's reported by Tischkoff. In addition, they found an additional SNP (-14,009 G) showing a strong statistical association with lactase persistence. In vitro studies indicated that this SNP altered lactase promoter binding in a manner similar to the -14,010 C SNP, providing a molecular confirmation of an effect on lactase. However, several subjects carrying the 14,009 G SNP proved to be lactase non-persistent in the breath hydrogen test. The authors speculated that this SNP may act less efficiently than the previously known persistence SNP's. Interestingly, these researchers found that all five known lactase persistence SNP's were present in their sample of Ethiopian students. Ethiopia is adjacent to Asia, and this region has often been a crossroads of human migration. This, in combination with the natural selection provided by dairying, underlies this diversity of lactase persistence. A subsequent report by Swallow and collaborators demonstrated that the -14009 G allele is also present in populations in the Sudan.[91] If this SNP is truly less efficient in amount of lactase produced, this could account for its low population penetrance.

The -13910 T allele (recall, this is the only allele found in traditional European populations) is not widespread in Africa, but it was found at a frequency of 27% in the Mozabite people of Algeria, and at lower frequencies in Arabic-related populations in the more southern countries of Cameroon and Chad. Given the proximity of Algeria to Europe and the Middle East, -13910 T may have been introduced from these areas, and haplotype analyses indicate both of these regions may have contributed this allele. Certainly this SNP traveled a long ways from its origin in central Europe, perhaps surfing the wave of spreading use of dairy.

The story of lactase persistence in Africa may be even more complicated than is indicated by the complex geographic distribution of these SNPs. In their study at Penn on diversity of African persistence, Dr. Ranciero and colleagues performed lactose tolerance tests on 322 individuals in their test population. Numerous lactase persistent Africans did not carry any of the known persistence SNPs. The authors hypothesized that other genetic mechanisms could account for lactase persistence, or that these individuals may possess an upper gut flora that allows them to consume lactose and develop elevated blood glucose levels, which was the diagnostic criterion for persistence in their variation of the lactose tolerance test. Similarly, the previously described research on Ethiopian college students also revealed several individuals who did not carry one of the known persistence SNP's, but who were still phenotypically lactase persistent. These populations await additional research.

LACTASE PERSISTENCE ON THE ARABIAN PENINSULA

Lactase persistence is common among the peoples of the Arabian Peninsula, reflecting a long dependence on dairy animals. Imtiaz and colleagues in Riyadh, Saudi Arabia, sequenced DNA from 432 blood samples collected from newborns in geographically diverse regions of Saudi Arabia.[92] They determined that the primary lactase persistence allele was -13,915 T, which as noted previously probably arose in this area about 4000 years ago. In addition, two individuals carried the -13,910 T allele, the predominant European allele. The overall incidence of genetic lactase persistence in individuals from these Saudi regions varied from 47% to 62%.

The following map summarizes the distribution of persistence SNP's in Africa and the Arabian Peninsula.

Distribution of Lactase Persistence SNP's in Africa and the Arabian Peninsula

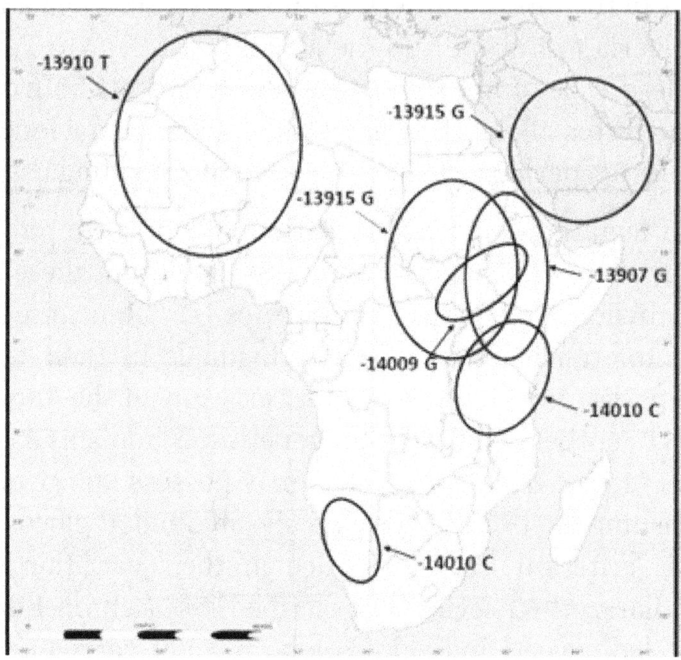

Figure 5: Constructed from references cited in this section. The shown distributions are conceptual constructions based on limited data. Some of these SNP's are only present in portions of the indicated area, and others may be more widely present than indicated.

LACTASE PERSISTENCE IN INDIA

India is the world leader in total dairy production, with both cattle and water buffalo serving as sources of milk. The appearance of lactase persistence here accompanied the exploitation of dairy. In addition to its spread throughout Europe and parts of Africa by migrating populations, migrating humans also carried the - 13,910 T SNP from central Europe eastward to the subcontinent of India. This allele is now widespread in India, likely the result of an Indo-Aryan migration from central Europe or western Asia. A study by Dr. Janaki Babu and colleagues in Lucknow and Bangalore determined that in northern India, where this Aryan genetic background is more common, 33% of the population carries this SNP for persistence. In contrast in Southern India, with less Aryan heritage, only 13% carried this SNP.[93] These investigators also tested their 153 volunteers for three of the SNP's discovered in Africa (-13,915 G, -14,009 G, and -14,010 C). No carriers were found. Therefore the considerable penetration of lactase persistence in India, particularly the north, appears to have arisen entirely from peoples migrating from the west.

DID THE -13,910 T SNP EVOLVE INDEPENDENTLY IN CENTRAL ASIA?

Lactase persistence is also present in much of central Asia. Evelyne Heyer and colleagues in Paris used DNA sequencing to determine the frequency of the - 13910 T allele over a large swath of central Asia including Kazakhstan and incorporating portions of the ancient Silk Road, which transported goods between the Eastern and Western worlds (and likely transported human genes as well).[94] The incidence of lactase persistence among the various populations varied somewhat; among Tajiko-Uzbek individuals, the incidence was 10%, compared to 17% for the Kazakh population. Given that a major overland trade route once passed through this area, it is reasonable to suspect this trait appeared through introgression from a European source. However, it is unclear whether the -13910 T allele in Central Asia does indeed share a common origin with the European gene. The authors determined that individuals carrying -13910 T tended to a have a low portion of a western-type gene pool, raising the possibility of an independent origin in Central Asia. Also, at the apparent time of origin of this allele, the Central Asian groups were culturally different from European farmers and pastoralists. They were nomadic, and their primary access to dairy was mare's milk. Interestingly, out of 183 Kazakh subjects in the study, a single individual was found to carry the -14010 C allele, which is widespread in populations of Eastern and Southern Africa. This suggests that some lactase persistence may arise from introgression, and further demonstrates the mingling of human genes facilitated by footloose individuals. Alternatively the single appearance of the -14010 C SNP could have also resulted from a rare mutation in peoples of this Eurasian plain.

More recent research supports a novel origin of -13,910 T in central Asia, rather than a transfer from Europe. A large consortium of researchers led by Dr.

Leena Peltonen in Helsinki (the team that was the original discoverers of the persistence SNP) identified four haplotypes containing the -13,910 T SNP in west Asia and far eastern Europe that appear to be quite distinct from the -13,910 T haplotype found in Europe and northern Africa.[95] Recall from the earlier discussion on genetics that diversity within haplotypes gradually increases due to mutations that accumulate over succeeding generations. The accumulated changes are used to estimate the length of time since different haplotypes diverged from a common ancestor. Peltonen and colleagues used this tool to determine the approximate age of these haplotypes. All four haplotypes in this region of western Asia and eastern Europe are fairly recent in origin, first appearing in populations of that area about 1,400 to 3,000 years ago. The same analysis indicates that the more common western European version of the -13,910 T SNP haplotype appeared between 5,000 and 12,000 years ago, corroborating the available archeological data. Many of the peoples of the steppes covering much of western Asia were traditionally herders, though they may have engaged in seasonal agriculture. This work indicates that this persistence SNP appeared de novo in these populations fairly recently, and its selective power has allowed it to spread into these pastoral dairy societies. Although persistence in this region may be the result of introgression from Europe, the current data indicate a strong possibility of local origin.

Tibet is another region where some individuals are lactase persistent. Genome sequence data indicate that Tibetan farmers domesticated yaks a little more than 7000 years ago, and Tibet has a long tradition of dairy based on yak milk.[96] A group associated with the Chinese Academy of Sciences reported that about one-third of contemporary Tibetans appear to be lactose tolerant based on a breath hydrogen test. Genetic tests by this group found that the five known persistence SNP's are not present in Tibetans at any appreciable frequency. However, they did find three unique SNP's in this area of the chromosome 2.[97] Unfortunately, there was no attempt to correlate the presence of these SNP's with ability to digest lactase. Obviously more work is needed to determine if a novel genetic change for persistence exists in this population.

SUMMARY OF DISTRIBUTION OF LACTASE PERSISTENCE SNP's

To complete our discussion, the lack of lactase persistence in most of the rest of the world must be noted. This represents the situation before European colonial expansion and the spread of the European version of the -13,910 T SNP. For example, lactase persistence appears to be very uncommon in China. In a recent genetic study of 120 individuals in Zhejiang Province, none of them had any of the known SNPs for adult lactase persistence.[98] Lactase persistence is similarly uncommon in the populations in the remainder of eastern Asia, as well as the original inhabitants of Americas, Australia, Pacific Islands, and many parts of Africa.

The following figure summarizes the distribution of lactase persistence SNP's in major geographic areas.[99]

Distribution of SNP's and Lactase Persistence in the Old World

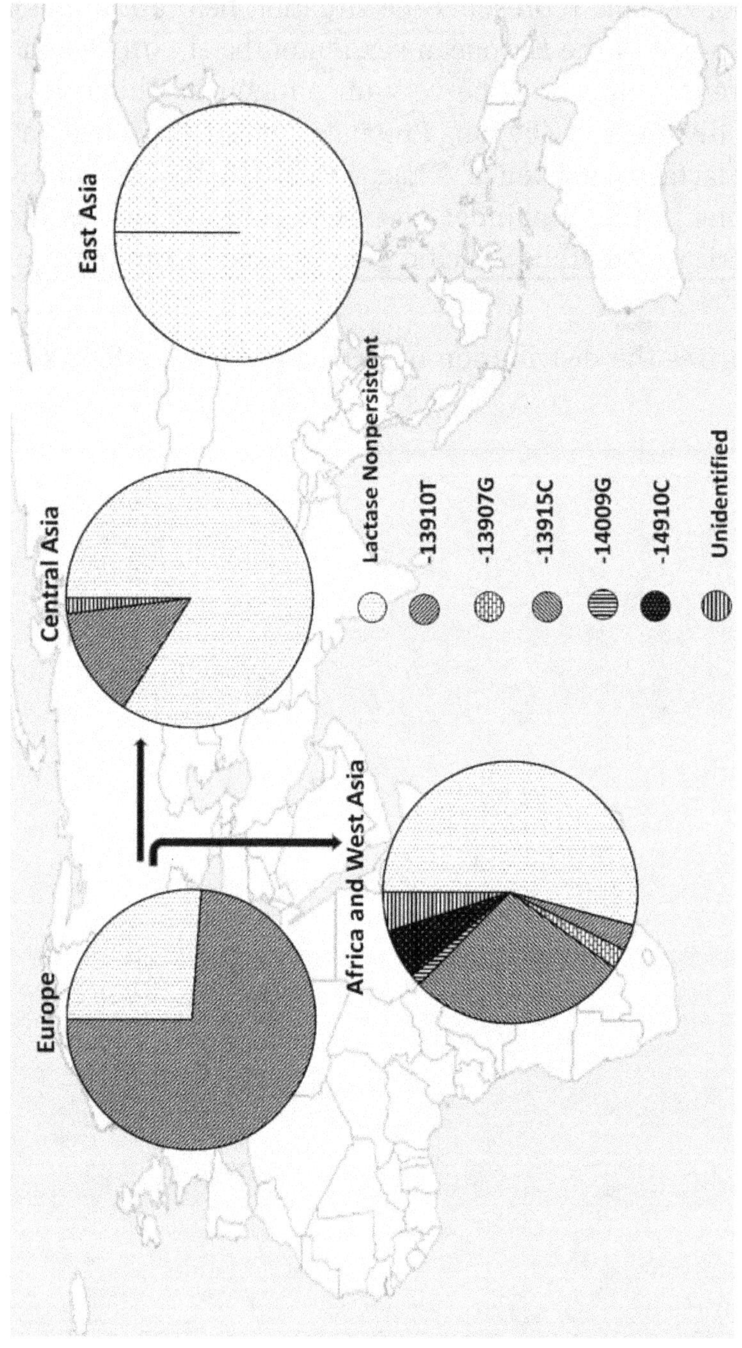

Figure 6: **Modified from DM Swallow and JT Troelsen, Nature Structural and Molecular Biology, 23:506 (2016).** Relative proportions of SNP's and extents of lactase persistence are approximate, and generally based on limited amounts of data and imprecise diagnostic assays (such as the hydrogen breath test). Arrows indicate that the -13910T SNP may have originated in Europe and spread to Asia and Africa by human migration. "Unidentified" indicates apparent lactase persistence that is not associated with a known SNP.

This chart strikingly highlights the extensive genetic diversity of lactase persistence in Africa, in comparison to other regions. Noteworthy is the size of the sector of "unidentified" lactase persistence in Africa. This is based on individuals who appear to be lactase persistent based on breath hydrogen tests, but do not carry one the known SNP's for lactase persistence. These tests are an imperfect measure of lactase persistence. However, the proportion of "unexplained" persistence is much higher in Africa, compared to Europe or Asia. This suggests that other genetic mechanisms for lactase persistence aside from the known SNP's may exist in African populations. Perhaps an interesting genetic mechanism still awaits discovery.

LACTASE PERSISTENCE IS BUT ONE EXAMPLE OF EVOLUTIONARY ADAPTATION TO DIETARY CHANGES

The development of lactase persistence in cultures that maintained dairy animals is just one example of how dietary changes and the accompanying natural selection have led to alterations in the human genome. These changes have been occurring among our forebears for millions of years, and have allowed humans to shift from a diet of raw meat and foraged plants to the modern diet of cooked meat, intensive consumption of starchy grains and root crops, and dairy.

Another example is duplications of the gene for salivary amylase production. Amylase is the digestive enzyme that breaks starch down into short glucose chains, which are further degraded to glucose by other enzymes.[100] This gene was duplicated, that is, a second copy appeared, early in human evolution. Amylase has undergone even more duplications in societies dependent on farming of starchy foods. For example in Japan, long reliant on rice, some individuals have 15 copies of the amylase gene, and 70% of the population has at least six copies. In contrast, in the Yakut, a Central Asian society based on herding and fishing, only 37% have six or more copies of amylase. In the grain dependent populations, increased copy number of the amylase gene allowed greater production of the enzyme, and individuals with more enzyme capacity apparently had a selective advantage because of an ability to obtain greater nutritional value from starchy food. This selective advantage may have been particularly important during times of famine or GI infections.

Starch digestion by man's best friend provides a parallel example of adaptation to the human diet. The first animal domestication was the development of dogs from wolves. Intentional domestication may not have occurred; rather humans and wolves may have lived in proximity, and selection for wolves that were more disposed to associate with humans may have led to the domestic dog. Wolf domestication occurred between 11,000 and 40,000 years ago, and long preceded human development of agriculture and domestication of ruminants. The genetic changes that improved accommodation to new diets in humans also occurred in dogs. This includes an improved ability to digest starch.[101] Wolves have two copies of a gene for pancreatic amylase. In comparison dogs have from four to as many as thirty copies of this gene, indicating multiple duplications after domestication. Because of this duplication, the levels of expression of this gene in the dog pancreas is up to 28 times that in the wolf pancreas. This increase in amylase copy number is most pronounced in dogs from areas that developed agriculture, which includes most temperate parts of the globe. Australia and the Arctic are areas where humans did not practice agriculture, and dogs native to these areas have fewer copies of the amylase gene. This suggests that an increase in amylase was not part of the original domestication of wolves, but developed later in dogs that lived in agricultural societies.[102] In comparison to wolves, dogs also have increased expression of the gene for maltase (this enzyme cleaves starch fragments produced by amylase into glucose). Additionally there is increased expression in dogs of an enzyme known as sodium/glucose linked cotransporter 1 (SGLT-1), which facilitates absorption of glucose from the intestine. This change allows dogs to more completely utilize glucose released during starch digestion. The increased activities of maltase and SGLT-1 are apparently due to both increased activity of the proteins involved in glucose uptake and an increase in their production due to gene duplication.

One can readily visualize these early dogs, with tails wagging, patiently begging tasty scraps of bread or less appealing droppings of whole grain porridge from their human masters. The dogs best able to digest the starch-rich diet had a strong selective advantage over their less fortunate littermates. Dogs had an advantage over humans in the pace of adapting to the starchy diet of early farming societies. A dog generation is about 2-4 years, compared to a human generation of 15-35 years. This combined with large litter sizes may have allowed more rapid selection of beneficial genetic changes in the dog gene pool.

The occurrence of multiple genetic changes in starch digestion suggests that a powerful genetic selection drove the dog's ability to thrive on a starchy human diet. The ability of dogs to fully digest bread (or other starchy foods) results from multiple genetically based physiological changes that likely developed over thousands of years. In contrast, the human change to lactase persistence required only a single minor genetic change, and the first full-fledged lactose tolerant individual emerged quite suddenly. It is worth noting that mature dogs appear to be uniformly lactase non-persistent, though this area has received little attention. Perhaps milk and dairy was not a selective factor for canines.

Lactase persistence is the best-documented case study of human adaptation to dietary changes. However, the changes in lactase and amylase mirror other changes that had occurred much earlier as humans tamed fire and transitioned from a diet of raw to cooked meat. Analyses of gene expression patterns indicate the magnitude of these changes. Researchers adapted mice to a carnivorous diet of raw or cooked organic beef eye round roast. After allowing the mice to become accustomed to this diet, they compared the expression patterns of liver enzymes in mice consuming raw versus cooked beef (well done).[103] Expression of numerous enzymes changed on the basis of whether the meat was raw or cooked. This indicated the enzymes that were upregulated in digesting raw or cooked beef, respectively. DNA sequences of the analogous genes in humans and chimpanzees (among our closest living ancestors) were compared. Many of the differentially expressed genes for cooked beef in mice have human analogs that are altered versus those of chimpanzees, which do not have access to cooked meat. This indicates that a human diet of cooked meat has resulted in natural selection of genetic changes that were beneficial for those consuming this new diet.

The human genome is not static. Rather, it is constantly changing in response to new selective forces arising from alterations in diet and lifestyle. The story of lactase persistence is probably the best understood of the known alterations of the genome in response to a changing environment.

7 DIAGNOSIS OF LACTOSE MALDIGESTION (AND LACTASE DIGESTION)

The previous chapters chronicled the widespread occurrence of genetic changes that result in adult lactase persistence. Despite these, about 70-80% of the world's population does not produce significant lactase after childhood, and these individuals may incur lactose malabsorption and perhaps intolerance symptoms after dairy consumption (particularly milk). Much of the remainder of this book explores the consequences of lactose intolerance, and the measures available for dealing with it. This chapter examines the procedures that are currently used for diagnosis, and provides a critical comparison of these methods. In particular, this chapter will help readers with suspected lactose intolerance or health care workers to understand the diagnostic options that are available, and what the test results mean.

DEFINITIONS: LACTOSE MALABSORPTION AND LACTOSE INTOLERANCE

Before exploring the diagnostic procedures, it is important to review definitions for lactose malabsorption and lactose intolerance. Clear definitions are essential for interpretation of test results.

A sharp distinction separates the seemingly similar terms "lactose malabsorption" and "lactose intolerance." "Lactose malabsorption" refers to the general inability of the small intestine to break down lactose and absorb the component sugars before lactose reaches the colon. In this condition, large amounts of lactose reach the colon intact. Malabsorption may occur because of a genetic shutdown of lactase production in the small intestine, or because of other factors that prevent lactose digestion even in the presence of the genetic ability to produce lactase.

"Lactose intolerance" refers to the symptomatic state that occurs in lactose malabsorbers when substantial lactose reaches the colon, causing the characteristic problems of gas, flatulence, distension, cramping, and diarrhea. Thus lactose intolerance occurs as a consequence of lactose malabsorption, but some individuals with lactose malabsorption do not experience these intolerance symptoms after dairy consumption.

The diagnosis of lactose intolerance can be complicated due to its multiple potential causes. As discussed in earlier chapters, most of the world's population lacks one of the SNPs that causes lactase production to continue into adulthood. Most of these individuals will likely experience some level of symptoms after sufficient amounts of dairy intake, with the symptom intensity varying based on intakes of other foods, activity and stress levels, and perhaps many other factors. Even individuals who do carry one of the SNPs for lactase persistence may experience symptoms of intolerance under certain conditions, a condition known as secondary lactose intolerance. Also, some individuals pass through most of adulthood with lactase persistence, but develop symptoms of intolerance with age. This age-related decline in ability to digest lactose in poorly understand. It is unclear whether this partial or total loss of lactase digestion is due to changes in gene expression that decrease the amount of enzyme, or some aging process in the villi and microvilli that causes loss or weakening of the cells that normally produce lactase. A later chapter explores secondary lactose intolerance in more detail.

Two varieties of diagnostic tests are available. The first are recently developed genetic tests that determine the presence of the DNA changes (SNPs) that confer adult lactase persistence. The second group are biochemical and physiological assays that measure the enzyme directly or the physiological responses to the ingestion of pure lactose (or sometime milk). Results of these tests do not necessarily align with genetic test results, and an individual who is genetically able to produce lactase in adulthood may still test as a lactose malabsorber. Similarly, someone who receives results of a genetic test indicating nonpersistence may still be able to consume dairy without the typical symptoms of lactose intolerance. A table at the end of this chapter provides a ready comparison of these various tests.

GENETIC TESTS

Genetic tests directly detect persistence SNP's. This straightforward approach does not inflict discomfort or lengthy time demands on the individual. This is in marked contrast to the biochemical and physiological tests discussed later, which may require fasting, multiple blood draws, and confinement to the lab or clinic for several hours. The genetic test typically begins with inserting a swab into the mouth and rubbing it over the interior surface of the cheek. This collects epithelial cells on the swab, which is placed in a carrier solution that protects the DNA in the cells. A laboratory then extracts DNA from the cells and amplifies it with the polymerase chain reaction (PCR). Some tests even dispense with the cheek swab, and a small snip of hair serves as the source of DNA. Still other test procedures use a tube of blood collected by venipuncture; this has the benefit of minimizing contamination with extraneous DNA. Regardless of the source, the amplified DNA is then hybridized with short "probe" DNA sequences that contain the matching base pair sequences for the DNA region of one of the SNPs responsible for lactase persistence. "Hybridization" refers to a process in which two strands of DNA having regions of matching base pairs, such as adenine and cytosine, or thymidine and guanosine, pair up with each other. If the probe contains a sequence that matches the DNA sequence (i.e. complementary DNA) of the individual, it forms a double stranded DNA structure that can be isolated and measured. Thus an individual whose DNA sample forms such a double strand with the SNP-bearing probe is lactase persistent. Under appropriate conditions DNA hybridization assays are exquisitely specific and the difference of a single base will determine whether a double-stranded DNA section forms. Typically the test is designed to detect the -13,910 SNP that is most common in European and west Asian populations.

Prometheus Laboratories in San Diego developed the first DNA test for lactase persistence in the United States in the early 2000's. This assay utilized a patent issued to Dr. Leena Peltonen and colleagues in Finland who first discovered this lactase persistence SNP. Other laboratories have developed similar tests. Although the initial test was limited to the -13910 T SNP, improvements in some of these tests have led to inclusion of all of the five currently known lactase persistence SNPs. In the United States, no genetic lactase test that has been approved by the Food and Drug Administration. However, clinical laboratories can develop their own tests (sometimes known as "home brew" tests) and sell these as a service. A physician or other medical professional must generally order these tests. These tests are considered "investigational," and insurance coverage may be problematic. Access to genetic testing is easier in some other countries. For example, in the United Kingdom, consumers can buy lactase test kits for submitting cheek swab samples to a central laboratory, with results forwarded directly to them.

Rapid advancement of DNA tests for ancestry and genealogy are rendering obsolete specific test kits for lactase non-persistence. 23andme®, one of the major players in the DNA ancestry business, now includes the lactase persistence European SNP locus (-13,910 T) as part of its standard test. Unfortunately, at the time of this writing, the other four known SNP's were not included. Hopefully this case of cultural imperialism will be resolved in the future. In a broader sense, consumer-directed DNA testing may provide individuals with insights into other issues of diet and digestion, as well as identifying remote relatives with whom they may have absolutely nothing in common (except some DNA sequences).

Interpretations of genetic test results for persistence must be nuanced. If an individual does not carry one of the SNP's for lactase persistence, that person may likely suffer some symptoms of lactose intolerance if large amounts of dairy products, especially milk, are consumed. Their gut bacteria may metabolize lactose in such a manner that symptoms are averted at low levels of lactose ingestion, but higher levels may overcome the gut bacteria's protective abilities. Thus a test showing an absence of the persistence SNPs should be a caution about extensive dairy consumption, and may serve as an explanation for previously experienced GI symptoms.

If test results demonstrate that a person does have one of the SNPs for persistence, this indicates that the individual has the genetic potential to produce lactase, and intolerance symptoms generally should not occur. However, some genetically persistent individuals may still experience symptoms of lactose intolerance (secondary lactose intolerance). A number of GI conditions that damage or destroy the tips of the intestinal villi where lactase is located may cause this. This secondary lactose intolerance may be chronic, or episodic as the underlying cause waxes and wanes. One benefit of a positive genetic test for lactase persistence is that it helps rule out genetically determined lack of lactase as the cause for dairy digestion problems, and suggesting that other GI issues may be responsible. Additional medical testing may be needed to discover the underlying cause.

BIOCHEMICAL TESTS

Several biochemical tests may be used to diagnose lactose malabsorption. One, intestinal biopsy, directly measures lactase levels in tiny tissue samples collected from the duodenum or jejunum (the first sections of the small intestine). The other tests are indirect and measure the metabolic products of lactose, either the component sugars (glucose and galactose), or the fermentation products of lactose produced by the colon bacteria. The following sections consider each of these tests.

INTESTINAL BIOPSY

Testing of biopsy samples collected during GI endoscopy has long been considered the gold standard for measuring lactase activity.[104] However, the invasive nature of the test generally limits its use to individuals suffering serious disease. Diagnosis of GI problems often involves endoscopy, and collection of tissue biopsies is frequently part of this procedure. An endoscope is threaded down the esophagus, through the stomach, and into the duodenum. A cutting device in the endoscope removes small snips of the intestinal lining. These tissue fragments may contain the villi that can produce lactase. A staining procedure detects any lactase activity in the biopsies. In this procedure, the biopsy is incubated with a colorless analog of lactose that contains an attached group (a chromophore) that is colorless when part of this analog, but becomes highly colored after it is released by lactase. Thus if lactase is present, this chromophore is released resulting in an intense color. Recently, a Finnish company (Biohit) developed a test kit for immediately testing biopsy samples in the physician's office, eliminating the wait for lab results. This test is currently available in Europe and Latin America, but not in the United States. Expression of lactase in the duodenum of even healthy, lactase persistent individuals may be spotty, and a clear determination of whether an individual is lactase persistent usually requires multiple samples.

LACTOSE CHALLENGE TESTS

The other common diagnostic procedures are variations of the lactose challenge test, which involve drinking a lactose solution (usually lactose dissolved in water with a little flavor) and measuring the physiological effects of lactose absorption or non-absorption. The use of a lactose solution instead of milk or dairy products helps to standardize the test procedure, avoids issues with the perishable nature of milk, and eliminates GI problems that could result from the fat or protein content of milk. These tests require the consumption of a very large amount of lactose. The standard protocol is 50 grams of lactose, which is roughly equivalent to the amount of lactose in a quart of milk. Some variations of the procedure only require 25 grams of lactose. For pediatric populations or individuals with low body weight, the lactose load is sometimes reduced to one gram per kilogram of body weight. The 50 gram test has been criticized as being excessive because it is far beyond what is associated with normal dairy intake. Not surprisingly, the patient may suffer considerable discomfort from the symptoms experienced during the procedure. A doctor's office or medical laboratory may not be a pleasant environment for enduring this ordeal. Two variants of this test will be examined below: (1) the blood glucose test, and (2) the breath hydrogen test. Sometimes physicians use these tests in combination, since both can be performed after a single ingestion of lactose.

BLOOD GLUCOSE TEST

The glucose test for lactose digestion is somewhat analogous to the glucose tolerance test used to diagnose diabetes. A key difference is that the glucose tolerance test requires drinking a solution of glucose, whereas the lactose malabsorption test involves lactose.

If an individual has sufficient intestinal lactase, it almost completely cleaves lactose into glucose and galactose. Both of these sugars are quickly absorbed into the bloodstream (unlike lactose, which is too large to be absorbed to a significant extent). Analysis of blood samples taken at time intervals measures the spike in blood glucose resulting from its release from lactose. A baseline blood sample is drawn before the patient drinks the lactose solution, and additional samples are collected every 15-30 minutes over a period of up to three hours. The glucose values are graphed to provide the overall curve of glucose absorption. Similar to the glucose tolerance test, this test must be performed after a period of fasting (typically at least eight hours) to avoid the elevations in blood glucose levels caused by food consumption, particularly carbohydrate intake. Generally, an increase in blood glucose of greater than 20 mg/dl at any time after drinking the lactose solution is considered diagnostic of lactase persistence. This indicates that an individual is unlikely to suffer symptoms of lactose intolerance.

Blood glucose levels can be affected by many factors aside from food intake. These include stress, time of day, and activity level. In order for the blood glucose test to be accurate in the presence of possible background interferences, enough lactose must be ingested to produce a robust and measurable blood glucose spike in lactase persistent individuals. This underlies the use of a lactose challenge of 50 grams. However, results from the 50 gram dose can be criticized for overstating the true incidence of lactose intolerance. For example, in a clinical trial by Dr. Noel Solomons and associates in Guatemala, some subjects classified as lactose intolerant based on the 50 g lactose challenge were still able to consume 12.5 g of lactose, equal to eight ounces of milk, without any symptoms.[105] However, use of lower levels of lactose in this test would compromise accuracy because the decreased elevation of glucose from lactose would be difficult to distinguish from normal background fluctuations. The 50 g lactose challenge has remained the standard test.

It is important to consider the other outcome of the test; that is, the lactose challenge does not produce an increase in blood glucose. If an individual is a malabsorber, ingested lactose will pass into the large intestine without being broken down into the component sugars. Hence in this test the absence of a significant increase in blood glucose is indicative of lactose malabsorption.

BREATH HYDROGEN TEST

Human metabolism does not produce hydrogen gas, and it is not normally a part of the atmosphere. The only source of hydrogen in the human body and in the air exhaled from the lungs is the fermentation of carbohydrates by colon microorganisms.[106] The lactose breath hydrogen test measures this gas in exhaled air. The abundant bacteria in the colon quickly ferment lactose, and production of copious amounts of hydrogen can occur soon after lactose ingestion by a person lacking lactase. Some individuals harbor intestinal bacterial populations that produce methane in addition to hydrogen, or more rarely entirely methane. Much of the hydrogen and methane produced in the colon is expelled as flatus, causing an embarrassing symptom of lactose intolerance. However, some of the hydrogen and methane is absorbed across the lining of the intestine and dissolves in the blood passing through the vessels surrounding the colon. When this blood reaches the lungs, the process of diffusion releases these dissolved gasses into the expired air, along with the carbon dioxide in the blood that results from normal metabolism. A gas chromatograph measures levels of these gases in samples of exhaled breath collected in a syringe or plastic bag.

Many small carbohydrates (monosaccharides or disaccharides) that are undigestible by human enzymes will generate hydrogen upon reaching the colon. This has given rise to a number of breath hydrogen tests for diagnosing GI disorders; the test for lactose is just one of these. These tests use fructose, xylose, and lactulose, in addition to lactose.[107] These tests can not only determine the digestibility of various sugars, but also measure the time between ingesting a material and its entry into the colon (known as upper GI transit time). Lactulose, a sugar somewhat similar to lactose, is not digested by any human enzyme, but colon bacteria rapidly ferment it. The time between drinking a lactulose beverage and onset of a major breath hydrogen peak is often used to measure upper GI transit time.

This lactose breath hydrogen test is probably the most common diagnostic for lactose malabsorption due to its relative simplicity (no blood draws are required), and it is typically performed in a medical clinic. After drinking a lactose solution, the patient periodically exhales into a plastic bag or tube, and the expired air is injected into a simple, portable gas chromatography apparatus to measure the hydrogen level.

This test is straightforward, but the patient must prepare. Dietary fiber and undigested starch are also fermented in the colon to yield hydrogen and methane, and for the most accurate result the patient should avoid consuming high fiber foods (including many fruits and vegetables) as well as starchy foods for at least one day before the test. The patient must also refrain from smoking before the test, as this interferes with hydrogen measurement. The patient must not have been treated with antibiotics for several weeks before the test, since they strongly disrupt the bacterial flora of the colon and may distort normal hydrogen production.

As in the blood glucose test, the breath hydrogen test begins with the patient drinking a beverage containing 25-50 grams of lactose. A baseline (before lactose ingestion) breath hydrogen sample determines any background hydrogen production. The clinic performs additional measurements at 10 to 20 minute intervals for up to three hours. Generally an increase in breath hydrogen levels of more than 20 ppm above the baseline indicates lactose malabsorption. Someone whose hydrogen level never exceeds this value is presumed to have effective levels of intestinal lactase. Lactose malabsorbers generally experience increases of much more than 20 ppm, and frequently over 100 ppm. As with the blood glucose test, during the test procedure patients may record the occurrence and severity of symptoms they are experiencing. Paradoxically, some individuals lacking lactase do not develop elevated hydrogen levels. A later section discusses possible reasons for this.

The test conditions can raise issues about its validity. As noted earlier, ingestion of 50 grams of lactose greatly exceeds normal dietary intake. However, decreasing the lactose load decreases the sensitivity of the test; that is, the ability of the test to identify bona fide lactose malabsorbers. In addition, many individuals who generate elevated hydrogen after the 50 g challenge are nonetheless able to consume cup quantities of milk (about 12 g of lactose) without suffering symptoms. A further criticism of use of a lactose solution is based on the observation that breath hydrogen levels are higher when a lactose solution is consumed in comparison to a similar amount of lactose in whole milk. Solomons determined that children consuming milk had breath hydrogen levels about 50% lower than when they consumed the same amount of lactose as a solution.[108] The fat and protein in milk slow stomach emptying. This spreads over a longer time the whole process of lactose reaching the colon and being fermented. The lactose in milk dribbles slowly into the colon, compared to the burst of lactose when consumed in the absence of fat and protein. This slow entry with milk consumption diminishes the peak hydrogen levels observed, and likely reduces symptom severity as well. A final caution is that if the subject did not adhere to the recommended diet on the day preceding the test, hydrogen produced from fiber and starch fermentation may cause a false positive result.

Methane production by some individuals is another complication. To maintain procedure simplicity and reduce equipment cost, generally only hydrogen is measured. For individuals who produce primarily methane from this fermentation, measuring only hydrogen could lead to an incorrect determination of lactose absorption. Even if methane is measured, low amounts in the breath could still lead to false negative results. Colonic methane results from bacteria reacting hydrogen with carbon dioxide to yield methane. Typically, a single molecule of methane is generated from four molecules of hydrogen, and this reaction causes a substantial reduction in gas volume. Other work combining the collection of gas directly from the colon with analysis of exhaled air from the same individual has demonstrated that many people produce methane in the colon, but it is not detectable in exhaled air.[109] This colonic methane may be directly expelled as flatus. Thus the absence of breath hydrogen or methane in some lactase deficient individuals may result from fermentation pathways that do not produce gas, or low level methane production that is not reflected in the exhaled air.

The lactase breath hydrogen test is based on an assumption that if functional levels of lactase are not present in the small intestine, then ingested lactose will pass intact into the colon, where its fermentation generates hydrogen. However, other recent work undermines the assumption that lack of lactase inevitably leads to the presence of hydrogen and possibly methane in the breath.

Researchers at the University of Leuven in Belgium used another procedure to learn more about the overall fate of lactose in the GI tract.[110] Carbon-13 (or ^{13}C) is a non-radioactive isotope of carbon that makes up about 1.1% of all carbon on Earth and carbon dioxide in the atmosphere (the remainder is almost entirely carbon-12 (^{12}C). Various plants differ in the ratio of ^{13}C to ^{12}C that they extract from the air during photosynthesis. In particular, the maize (corn) plant and its seeds are enriched in the ^{13}C:^{12}C ratio. This enrichment in ^{13}C carries across into products made from animals eating corn. Therefore, if lactose is purified from the milk of cows consuming a corn diet, this lactose has an elevated $^{13}C{:}^{12}C$ ratio.

An analytical instrument known as a mass spectrometer can measure this ratio in exhaled air with extreme accuracy, and this can determine how quickly a ^{13}C-enriched food is digested. The researchers at Leuven used ^{13}C-enriched lactose to tract the fate of lactose (and its component sugars) in a variation of the lactose breath hydrogen test. If functional levels of lactase are present, increased ^{13}C resulting from human metabolism of glucose and galactose derived from lactose appears in the breath very quickly after ingestion. This appearance of $^{13}CO_2$ in the breath is more rapid than hydrogen resulting from colonic lactose fermentation. This test differs from the approach of measuring exhaled hydrogen or methane in that it can quantitate the carbon dioxide arising from the human metabolism of the glucose and galactose enzymatically released from lactose. Thus it is a direct measure of the human metabolism of lactose.

The results of this Belgian research provide the surprising finding that in a substantial portion of people lacking functional levels of lactase there is no increase in production of breath hydrogen or methane after drinking the lactose challenge solution. Out of all the subjects in this study who were diagnosed with lactase deficiency based on low $^{13}CO_2$ breath excretion, 41% did not produce either breath hydrogen or methane after the lactose challenge. This suggests that in these individuals colonic fermentation is not metabolizing lactose via a pathway that leads to abundant gas production. Colonic microflora may be metabolizing lactose by non-gas generating processes that are less troublesome to the individual. This supports the colonic adaptation hypothesis, which is the idea that colonic microorganisms can adapt to more benign processes for fermenting lactose. The following chapter provides more information on adaptation in the context of treatment options.

ACCURACY AND COMPARABILITY OF TESTS FOR LACTASE PERSISTENCE AND LACTOSE MALABSORPTION

Since the introduction of genetic tests for the lactase persistence SNP, several investigators have compared genetic results with blood glucose and breath hydrogen tests. In a German study,[111] subjects received the breath hydrogen test, and were also tested for the -13,910 T SNP (by far the most common SNP in Germany). The agreement between the two tests was very strong, as 95% of the subjects with positive breath hydrogen levels had the -13,910 C/C genotype; that is, neither chromosome 2 copy contained the T lactase persistence SNP. However, two subjects had the -13,910 T SNP, but were breath hydrogen positive. One subject suffered from Crohn's Disease, with the condition in an active state at the time of the test. Crohn's Disease damages the villi of the small intestine, and the condition may have affected this individual's intestinal lactase production. A second individual with the -13,910 T SNP also had a positive breath hydrogen test, but the breath hydrogen level attained its peak at 20 minutes after lactose consumption, a must faster rise than normally occurs in breath hydrogen producers. The authors postulated that this individual had an overgrowth of bacteria in the small intestine (the normal small intestine has a very, very low population of bacteria). In an overgrowth situation like this, the bacteria can quickly attack the ingested lactose, and produce hydrogen even if normal lactase is present in the villi.

SUMMARY

Lactose intolerance is by definition the state of suffering from symptoms related to lactose malabsorption. All of the biochemical tests covered in this chapter evaluate malabsorption, not intolerance. Similarly, the genetic tests evaluate the ability of adults to produce lactase, and do not involve direct measurement of symptoms. Lactose intolerance is really a perception of symptoms, and basically a mental state not directly subject to physiological diagnosis. Not surprisingly, a review of studies using the breath hydrogen test found little correlation between diagnostic test results and self-reported GI symptoms or milk intolerance.[112]

Despite the described shortcomings, traditional breath hydrogen and blood glucose tests remain the most credible tools for determining if an individual has functional levels of lactase. If these tests indicate lactose malabsorption (a deficiency in lactase), this may arise from the individual not having the genetic potential for lactase persistence (i.e. lacking any of the five known SNP's). Alternatively, the individual may have one of these SNP's, but another GI issue is limiting lactase production leading to malabsorption. Here, the use of a genetic test would provide insight into the reason for observed malabsorption. The following table summarizes the previously discussed test procedures.

Table 3: Comparison of Tests for Lactose Malabsorption

Test	Technical Basis	Advantages	Disadvantages
Genetic	DNA hybridization used to detect presence of SNP for persistence	Non-invasive (if cheek swab is used)	Even if SNP for persistence is found, secondary intolerance may still be present. Test may be limited to the most common SNP (-13,910 T).
Intestinal biopsy	Detection of lactase in intestinal tissue	Considered "Gold Standard" for diagnosis.	Highly invasive and usually used only when a more serious condition is suspected. Multiple samples (collected at the same time) needed for accuracy.
Lactose challenge breath hydrogen	Excretion of hydrogen in the breath after colonic fermentation of lactose. Methane levels in breath may also be measured.	Probably most common test; prominent role in scientific literature.	Fasting required. Subject must remain in clinic for several hours. Prior food consumption may affect results. Methane production may reduce hydrogen excretion.
Lactose blood glucose challenge	Measures increase in blood glucose resulting from activity of intestinal lactase.	Perhaps more accurate than breath hydrogen.	Fasting required. Multiple blood draws; subject must remain in clinic for several hours. Food consumption or stress may also affect blood glucose.

8 THE DECLINE OF LACTASE DURING CHILDHOOD

The two previous chapters explored the genetics of adult lactase and the procedures used for diagnosis of persistence and nonpersistence. In individuals lacking one of the five SNP's for persistence, lactase declines inexorably during childhood. However, these chapters did not discuss the specific age of onset of lactase decline (or appearance of lactose malabsorption). This chapter explores this poorly understood area. This topic is important because it may shed light on digestive problems that may appear in children, particularly if the family history suggests a possibility of adult lactose malabsorption. It must be emphasized that the decline in lactase as children become older is difficult to measure, and likely subject to many sources of variation. Unfortunately, in comparison to the previous chapters there is a dearth of information about the age of onset.

ONSET OF LACTOSE MALABSORPTION IS GRADUAL, AND THE TOOLS FOR ITS MEASUREMENT IMPRECISE

As described in Chapter 4, epigenetic alterations of DNA appear responsible for the gradual shutdown of lactase production, and there is likely a "gray zone" during which lactase slowly declines and the concomitant symptoms of lactose intolerance begin. The imprecise nature of the available diagnostic tests (blood glucose and breath hydrogen assays) complicates the task of tracking how a child transitions from lactose absorber to a malabsorber. Differences in the performance of these tests add further uncertainty. Slight differences in protocols could sway whether an individual in this gray zone is diagnosed to have hypolactasia. This chapter summarizes the available data, with a caveat that the limited information does not permit strong conclusions.

Generally, an individual is assigned to absorber or malabsorber status based on specific breath hydrogen and blood glucose values. However, this binary approach does not reflect the actual human experience. Most likely, individuals with progressing malabsorption may begin to experience some symptoms after dairy consumption, with severity increasing with age. They may eventually stop consuming some dairy products, particularly if symptoms are severe. In addition, many individuals with malabsorption do not appear to suffer intolerance symptoms. These individuals may pass through childhood with lactase gradually declining, yet never suffer negative effects.

Another factor complicating interpretation of test results is the large amount of lactose used. Tests in children typically use two grams of lactose per kilogram of body weight.[113] A child undergoing a decline in lactase likely weighs about 15 to 40 kilograms, so they are consuming 30 to 80 grams of lactose (many studies limit consumption to a maximum of 50 grams). For perspective, a pint of milk contains about 24 grams of lactose. A child's limited remaining lactase may be unable to adequately digest this huge challenge, and they consequently fall into the malabsorption category. However, if they consumed a more normal amount of milk (such as an eight ounce cup with twelve grams of lactose), the remaining lactase could possibly break down this smaller amount. In addition, the lactose challenge test is performed with a lactose solution. This is definitely a worst case situation compared to normal dietary patterns, where the protein and fat in milk slow stomach emptying and intestinal transit, providing the remaining lactase more contact time with substrate. Additionally, consumption of dairy as part of a meal further slows GI passage.

With these caveats about diagnosing the condition in mind, we will cautiously review the limited research. An evaluation of the decline of lactase activity in Sardinian children provides insight into this age of onset issue.[114] Most Sardinians develop hypolactasia during childhood, as only about 10% of the population possesses the - 13910 T SNP for adult persistence. Enrico Schirru and colleagues in Cagliari, Italy performed breath hydrogen tests on 392 youths between the ages of 3 and 19. They also determined the -13,910 C/C genotype of these subjects (recall that this is the genotype associated with nonpersistence). Hypolactasia began to appear in some C/C individuals as early as 3-4 years of age, with 32% of this group having a positive breath hydrogen test. This trend progressed steadily to 41% at 5-6 years, 72% at 7 years, 86% at 8 years, and 93% at 9 years. Between 9 and 19, the percentage of youths with positive breath tests remained in the range of 93-95%. Thus, it appears that the shutdown of lactase appears to be uniform by age 9. Interestingly, there was a small portion (5-7%) of older youths who had negative breath hydrogen tests despite not having a persistence SNP. This supports the observation in the previous chapter that some individuals with hypolactasia are able to somehow metabolize lactose without significant hydrogen production. These researchers did not monitor methane levels, and possibly some of these atypical subjects excreted solely methane.

The Sardinian results indicate that a substantial loss of lactase occurs in some children as early as three or four, and this proportion increases with age. This study is unique in reporting the incidence of non-persistence at different ages in the same population. Other studies provide supporting data on non-persistence in children in other populations. Mexican-American children in Texas showed a similar trend in declining lactase with age.[115] In a group of children ranging in age from two to five (mean age of 4.7), 32% were lactase non-persistent based on breath hydrogen results. In a group of six to nine year olds (mean of 7.9), 40% were non-persistent. The oldest group tested was 10 to 14 years of age (mean of 10.4), and 56% were non-persistent. This level of non-persistence is similar to a separately reported level of 54% in Mexican-American adults.[116] Thus it appears that most Mexican-Americans who would become lactase non-persistent adults made this transition in their first decade. In both this study and the Sardinian investigation noted above, about 1/3 or more children were non-persistent before their fifth birthday, with many additional children becoming non-persistent by their tenth birthday. In both studies, virtually all individuals without SNP's for persistence lose an appreciable amount of their intestinal lactase in the first decade of life.

A few other studies provide insight into the age of onset in various populations. In early work, Drs. Garza and Scrimshaw at the Massachusetts Institute of Technology used various lactose tolerance tests to determine the incidence of intolerance (measured by overt symptoms) in black children in the

Boston area.[117] In a group of nine children aged four or five, only one developed symptoms. In contrast, 50% of a larger (24) group of six and seven olds were intolerant and this increased to 72% in a group of eight or nine year olds. The incidence in this final group is close to a value of 70% or more reported for black American adults.[118] Researchers at Johns Hopkins University examined malabsorption in black children in Baltimore, but evaluated only children less than five.[119] In the group of 116 children evaluated, 25% showed malabsorption in a lactose challenge test of two grams of lactose per kilogram of body weight. In a subgroup of 36 children between 12 and 23 months, nine were already lactose intolerant, based on a blood glucose test following lactose ingestion. However, the investigators used a blood increase of less than 26 mg/100 ml as a measure of lactose intolerance. Most investigators have used a threshold of less than 20 mg/100 ml, so the Baltimore results may overstate the incidence of intolerance in this young population.

With the exception of the Sardinian study, these investigations on malabsorption were performed prior to the availability of genetic tests. The absence of this information complicates using these data to evaluate the age when functional levels of lactase disappear, since children with a persistence SNP will continue producing lactase into adulthood. Although these prior studies were hampered by an inability to identify the children with genetic persistence, in several the incidence of malabsorption in nine or ten year olds closely reflected the adult incidence in these populations, suggesting that genetic changes causing hypolactasia are largely complete by this age.

Some scientists have speculated that the age of onset of hypolactasia varies among different regions or ethnic groups, although no available data support this viewpoint. In fact, the papers cited here indicate that this process begins universally at an early age, with substantial numbers of children in multiple ethnic groups with hypolactasia by five, and full conversion to adult primary hypolactasia state by nine or ten. Thus the childhood process of losing lactase appears to proceed inexorably based on genetics, uninfluenced by the environment.

Prior to humans domesticating milk-producing animals, there was no apparent functional role for lactase in any mammal after weaning, and evolutionary pressure for metabolic efficiency led to its shutdown early in life. However, this shutdown is gradual, and perhaps a slow shutdown even assists in the weaning process, with milk becoming less palatable to offspring. There is no substantiated involvement of environment or ethnicity in this shutdown, though future research may yield novel findings.

SUMMARY

Lactase production in non-persistent children gradually ceases. In some children, lactose malabsorption may appear in the second year of life; in others almost a full decade may pass before lactose malabsorption fully manifests itself. Regardless of age of onset, this cessation appears to be generally gradual. However, it is possible that severe intestinal infections, as are common in some undeveloped areas, could accelerate this shutdown. It is unknown if the rate of shutdown is under the influence of genetic or environmental factors. These intriguing questions await future research.

9 SECONDARY LACTOSE INTOLERANCE

SOME LACTOSE INTOLERANCE IS NOT DUE TO GENETICS

Most people who have inherited a SNP conferring adult lactase persistence go through life consuming dairy without ill effect. However, some eventually encounter the well-known symptoms of intolerance, a condition known as secondary lactose intolerance.

Our discussion to this point has focused on primary lactose intolerance, which develops after the gene for lactase shuts down during childhood. In contrast, secondary lactose intolerance is a condition that occurs in individuals who are genetically capable of producing lactase into adulthood, but who still lack functional lactase levels. This condition attracts relatively little attention. Perhaps this is because secondary lactose intolerance is often a consequence of very serious GI diseases, and the inability to consume dairy may be low on the lists of concerns for many of these patients. Despite lack of attention, secondary lactose intolerance may be quite common, particularly among the elderly. This chapter examines some of the causes of secondary lactose intolerance, the demographics of its sufferers, and possible ways to ameliorate this condition.

INFECTION AND INFLAMMATION AS CAUSES

As noted earlier, the cells lining the small intestine are located on hair-like protrusions known as villi that extend from the folds of the intestinal wall. These villi greatly increase the surface area of the intestine, and enormously increase its absorptive capacity. The very tips of the villi tend to be the sites of lactase activity. Illnesses that damage the villi tend to take a toll on the highly exposed villi tips, destroying lactase activity. This accounts for the frequent occurrence of lactose intolerance in diseases or conditions that damage the small intestine.

Celiac disease is often accompanied by lactose intolerance.[120] Celiac is an inflammation of the intestine caused by an immune response to gluten, a wheat protein. This inflammatory process damages the intestinal villi, and lactase production may be partly or completely lost. Treatment for celiac disease (usually a strict gluten-free diet) may eventually reverse the damage, restoring functional levels of lactase.

British researchers demonstrated this restoration of lactase after celiac disease was treated. They collected duodenal biopsies from celiac patients who were primarily of northern European ancestry and hence largely genetically lactase persistent.[121] The samples were assayed for lactase. Levels were normal in celiac patients without active disease. However, lactase was absent in those with active disease. It was restored in patients who had previously had active disease, but had been in remission for three months. Possibly celiac-induced lactose intolerance could contribute to the GI symptoms suffered by these patients. Fortunately, this loss of lactase activity in celiac appears to be a generally transitory phenomenon that disappears upon successful treatment.

Gluten sensitivity is a related but less severe condition. Little attention has been paid to the occurrence of secondary lactose intolerance in gluten sensitivity, and it is unclear if lactose intolerance contributes to the diffuse GI symptoms suffered by some gluten sensitive individuals. Similar to celiac disease, strict adherence to a gluten-free diet could gradually allow restoration of the enzyme and reverse lactose intolerance.

A difficult to diagnose condition known as small intestine bacterial overgrowth (or SIBO) is potentially a major cause of secondary intolerance. Symptoms of SIBO include bloating, abdominal pain, nausea, and diarrhea; all of these are somewhat similar to the symptoms of lactose intolerance and irritable bowel syndrome. It is more common in the elderly. The small intestine normally has a quite low population of bacteria, with the contents of the upper small intestine containing fewer than 1000 bacteria per milliliter.[122] This relatively low level of bacteria is due to a number of factors, including the acidity of the stomach that kills many of the bacteria ingested in food or drink, and the rapid passage of material from the stomach through the small intestine that allows little time for proliferation of surviving bacteria. In SIBO, the bacterial content of the intestine (measured in aspirates from the jejunum) is 1000 per milliliter or greater (often much greater).

SIBO has a multiplicity of possible causes, including slowed intestinal motility, celiac disease, certain immunological disorders, and surgical alterations of the intestine. Proton pump inhibitors, including such over-the-counter drugs as omeprazole and lansoprazole, strongly suppress the production of stomach acid. This is what makes them so effective against heartburn and acid reflux. However, frequent use of these drugs is associated with an increased incidence of SIBO,[123] demonstrating the importance of stomach acid in keeping the small intestine relatively clean of bacteria. At the other end of the small intestine, the ileocecal valve at the junction of the ileum and the colon prevents the reflux of the immense population of bacteria in the colon into the small intestine. Diverticular disease results from the development of pouches in the walls of the lower GI tract. It is more common in the elderly, and may impair normal peristalsis in the colon. This may permit colon bacteria to enter small intestine. Lactose intolerance is sometimes associated with diverticular disease, and treatment of this condition generally restores lactose tolerance.[124]

One source of SIBO symptoms is fermentation of digesta by the elevated bacterial population in the small intestine. The byproducts of this fermentation may include hydrogen gas, which can cause bloating, cramping, and other abdominal discomfort. In addition, the bacteria themselves or their byproducts may inflame the lining of the intestine. The body's own immune response to this bacterial insult may exacerbate the condition. This inflammation can affect absorption of nutrients, and it may damage the villi tips where lactase resides. The damage may be sufficient to render SIBO sufferers lactose intolerant, and furthermore the symptoms of lactose intolerance may exacerbate overall SIBO symptoms. More broadly, untreated SIBO may lead to forms of malnutrition arising from impaired digestion.

SIBO is difficult to diagnose, and two problematic approaches are commonly used. One approach is the microbiological testing of aspirates collected from the jejunum with a catheter, obtained by snaking it down the throat and through the stomach to reach the intestine. This test has poor reliability. Distribution of bacteria in the intestine may not be uniform, so testing of a single sample may not be representative. This procedure only retrieves samples from the upper small intestine, whereas SIBO may predominate in more distal areas of the intestine. In addition, the bacteria causing SIBO may not be readily cultured in the laboratory, particularly if they are anaerobic bacteria that entered from the colon through the ileocecal valve. Thus these lab cultures may produce false negatives. The time since food consumption and the composition of the meal may also affect the levels of bacteria in SIBO. This adds additional uncertainty. This microbiological testing of catheter samples is invasive and labor intensive, and infrequently used.

The other diagnostic test is a variation of the hydrogen breath tests often used to determine carbohydrate maldigestion. Lactulose is a synthetic sugar somewhat similar to lactose, but it is not broken down by intestinal lactase, and it is not usually absorbed. However, many bacteria readily ferment it. The lactulose challenge test consists of having a patient drink a solution of lactulose, and then measuring the concentration of hydrogen in the exhaled air at specific time intervals. If high levels of bacteria are present in the small intestine, they begin to ferment lactulose quickly after it leaves the stomach. However, lactulose is also fermented in the colon. This produces a separate later spike in breath hydrogen levels. The key factor in using the lactulose test for SIBO diagnosis is the rapidity of hydrogen production after lactulose consumption. Rapid onset of hydrogen indicates SIBO, and a slower response suggests normal colonic fermentation. One complication is that GI transit times differ greatly among people, and in someone with rapid transit, lactulose may quickly reach the colon and be fermented, yielding a false positive for SIBO. This variable related to transit time can be remedied by adding a radioactive isotope to the lactulose solution, and watching its passage through the small intestine and into the colon with gamma scintigraphy. However, this complex isotope approach involves exposure of the patient to radioactivity and requires the use of expensive equipment.

SIBO diagnosis may use other variants of the breath test. In one, glucose replaces lactulose. In normal individuals, glucose is rapidly absorbed in the small intestine. It is not fermented in the small intestine, and none enters the colon to be fermented to hydrogen. However, in individuals with SIBO bacteria ferment some glucose before it can be absorbed. This will result in an early burst in breath hydrogen. Sometimes a glucose test follows an initial positive lactulose test as a means for ruling out rapid intestinal transit as a cause for the lactulose result. A final variant is the use of lactose instead of lactulose. In SIBO, there will be early production of hydrogen as a result of intestinal fermentation. This approach is again compromised by the possibility of false positive results arising in individuals who are lactose intolerant and have rapid intestinal transit.

Of the two testing approaches, the first is prone to false negatives, and the second to false positives. Breath hydrogen tests yield greater prevalence rates for SIBO than do cultures of endoscopy samples.[125] Given the variability in the test procedures themselves and some differences in the diagnostic criteria for SIBO, it is not surprising that reported incidence rates vary widely. The reported range of incidence of SIBO for IBS patients varies from 4% to 64%.

Lactose intolerance is apparently more common in SIBO patients than in the underlying population. Investigators in northern Italy found 72% of SIBO patients to be lactose intolerant, compared to 6% in normal controls from the same population.[126] It was not possible to divide these cases of lactose intolerance into the portions caused by primary and secondary lactose intolerance. One of the treatments for SIBO is rifaximin, a non-absorbable oral antibiotic that is only effective in the GI tract. Treatment of a group of these Italian SIBO patients with a combination of rifaximin and a lactose-free diet resulted in a SIBO eradication rate of 98% (based on symptom reports), whereas only 32% of SIBO cases resolved in a second group treated with only a lactose-free diet. Unfortunately, the investigators did not test the individuals cured of SIBO for elimination of lactose intolerance. Definitive data on whether treatment for SIBO resolves lactose intolerance have yet to be developed. However, it seems clear that some incidences of secondary lactose intolerance arise from SIBO and these lactose-induced symptoms may actually contribute to the SIBO severity.

SECONDARY INTOLERANCE INCREASES WITH AGE

Aging tends to have adverse effects on the stomach and colon, and problems such as heartburn, indigestion, and constipation become more common in the elderly. In contrast, the small intestine appears quite well preserved during human aging.[127] However, the incidence of lactose intolerance increases in the later years, with some people who were once dairy digesters becoming lactose intolerant in their 50's, 60's, and 70's. This age-related increase is poorly recognized, and the reasons are largely unclear, but the increased incidence of GI issues such as SIBO undoubtedly play a role. Italian gastroenterologists evaluated the incidence of lactose malabsorption in the elderly.[128] In individuals younger than 65, about 58% were malabsorbers (this is to be expected for Italy, where the European adult lactase persistence trait is much less common than in northern Europe). In contrast, the incidence of malabsorption increased to about 83% in those older than 74. The group between 65 and 74 were intermediate, with about 63% malabsorbers. These results suggest that the likelihood of malabsorption increases rapidly as individuals pass their 70th birthdays. Interestingly, among the lactose malabsorbers in all three of these groups, the group over 74 experienced the lowest prevalence of lactose intolerance symptoms. The authors suggested that this decrease could arise from lowered pain perception in the elderly, or other alterations in nerve pathways. The authors apparently did not determine whether this population simply tended to avoid dairy products.

This increase in lactose intolerance with age, similar to many other conditions of aging, has attracted little research attention. Treatment approaches for secondary lactose intolerance in general are also unclear. Lactose-free dairy products and enzyme supplements should be effective. In addition, there are reports that some probiotic supplements are effective against SIBO. Perhaps the probiotic bacteria competitively displace the harmful bacteria in the intestine, or possibly the probiotics produce metabolites that eliminate them. Information for this application of probiotics is currently very limited, and the available studies are generally small and flawed in design. Obviously additional research is needed to understand the etiologies of secondary hypolactasia in the elderly (and others), and to determine effective treatment approaches.

SUMMARY

Infection or inflammation of the small intestine may cause secondary lactose intolerance, and its occurrence increases with age. An individual who suspects this condition may refrain from high-lactose dairy products to see if the condition resolves. Correcting the underlying condition may result in restoration of adequate intestinal lactase, though this recovery may be slow. Individuals suffering from secondary lactose intolerance can obtain immediate relief by consuming lactose-free dairy products or lactase supplements. In addition, probiotics may help some people in restoring normal intestinal function.

10 THE CHALLENGE OF LIVING WITH LACTOSE MALABSORPTION AND INTOLERANCE

THE LACTOSE INTOLERANT MAY FACE CONFUSING GUIDANCE

Those with lactose intolerance face sometimes difficult decisions on dairy consumption. They are rightly concerned about whether any dairy intake is advisable, or what quantities and types of dairy products they should consume. Recommendations are often confusing. There is even guidance that the lactose intolerant should force themselves to consume increasing amounts of milk, based on the hypothesis that the human body (or the body's intestinal microflora) will eventually adapt to metabolizing lactose in a friendlier manner, and symptoms will disappear. This chapter evaluates the frequent assertion that the lactose intolerant can consume some amount of milk (typically specified as one cup) without encountering any symptoms. Additionally it explores the diverse physiological mechanisms that allow some malabsorbers to consume substantial amounts of dairy, including milk, without ill effect. Finally, we will consider the "colonic adaptation" theory that ingestion of dairy or beneficial bacteria (probiotics) can decrease severity of lactose intolerance symptoms. Continuing the story, the next chapter covers several other approaches for treating lactose intolerance.

CHALLENGES IN CLINICAL EVALUATION OF TREATMENTS FOR LACTOSE INTOLERANCE

Well-designed clinical trials are essential for the critical evaluation of approaches for dealing with lactose intolerance. However, trials in this area have yielded results that are often conflicting or of questionable validity. Some appear to raise questions about whether milk consumption by malabsorbers even leads to symptoms. Entrenched camps of differing viewpoints in the scientific community and funding from various business interests have likely added to the commotion. The camp that downplays the significance of lactose intolerance conveys an implied message to the lactose intolerant population that their condition may not exist, or that the issue is largely just in their heads. However, those who suffer from lactose intolerance are quite aware that their condition is quite real, not imagined. They may strongly disagree with the "lactose intolerance denial approach" that some have pursued in the scientific literature.

Substantial technical difficulties complicate execution of clinical trials of treatments for lactose intolerance. Clinicians can diagnose lactose malabsorption with very objective measures such as elevated breath hydrogen or blood glucose. In contrast, lactose intolerance is by a definition an affliction of suffering symptoms after lactose ingestion. Any treatment purported to improve this condition must deliver a decrease in symptoms. Herein lies the pitfall. The target symptoms are quite subjective, and likely are affected by not only the GI response to lactose, but also the individual's overall health status, mood, and the ever present burden of problems that daily life presents. To further complicate the issue, the long-time sufferer of lactose intolerance (particularly the severe sufferer) may carry a psychological burden of past unpleasant experiences with dairy consumption. These experiences may trigger conditioned emotional and physiological responses to dairy consumption, regardless of whether the dairy product contains lactose. In some individuals with prior bad experiences, it is possible that dairy consumption will trigger stress reactions of diarrhea, increased GI motility, and cramping that are similar to those of bona fide lactose intolerance. In light of these concerns, it is not surprising that the generally small clinical trials in this area have frequently failed to show an effect of treatments on decreasing symptoms. An insightful example of these clinical trial difficulties and shortcomings is the observation that 100% lactose-free milk sometimes does not decrease intolerance symptoms, in comparison to consumption of similar quantities of milk containing a normal amount of lactose. [129] The lactose-free milk obviously cannot generate symptoms of lactose intolerance. The confusing outcomes of these trials likely lies in inadequate design, or the difficulties faced by subjects in distinguishing symptoms of true lactose intolerance from the psycho-physiological symptoms induced by a deeply ingrained history of bad experiences with dairy consumption. Perhaps one remedy for clinical trials of lactose-free dairy would be to conduct studies of a much longer duration (weeks or months), in comparison to past trials that have compared only a single ingestion of lactose-free milk with milk containing the full lactose load. A longer duration study might allow subjects receiving lactose-free milk to "unlearn" their conditioned behaviors, and recognize that the treatment that they are receiving is not burdened by imprinted symptoms. Subjects receiving lactose-containing milk would not experience this longer-term benefit.

LIMITED DATA SUPPORT THE "ONE CUP RULE"

As noted earlier, a frequent assertion is that lactose intolerant individuals can consume a limited amount of milk (usually stated as a cup, or eight ounces) without suffering any symptoms.[130] Generally this milk is suggested to be consumed with a meal. This "one cup rule" does not reflect the subtleties in individual responses to lactose intake, and perhaps variations in individuals over time. Only a few limited scale studies, some with questionable design, support this assertion. A proposal such as this that seeks to influence human nutrition should be supported by unequivocal data.

An example of the confusion in this area, and the attempt to draw firm conclusions from weak data, is the Consensus Statement issued by the National Institutes of Health (NIH) after the Consensus Conference on Lactose Intolerance in 2010.[131] The NIH convened a panel of experts to answer a number of questions related to lactose intolerance. One question involved how much lactose an individual with lactose malabsorption could consume without suffering symptoms. The panel opined: "The available evidence suggests that adults and adolescents with diagnosed lactose malabsorption could ingest at least 12 g of lactose when administered in a single dose (equivalent to the lactose content in 1 cup of milk) with no or minor symptoms." Note that this statement was an independent opinion of the panel, and was not a policy statement of the NIH. However, some sources have positioned this statement as an authoritative determination to support the idea that lactose intolerant individuals can consume significant amounts of dairy without ill effects. Given the imprimatur of credibility imparted to this statement by its association with the NIH, it is worth delving into the data used to support it.

The NIH panel drew upon a systematic review of the lactose intolerance literature developed by the Center for Evidence-Based Medicine at the University of Minnesota;[132] a government contract funded this work. The Center compiled all of the possibly relevant published clinical trials, but found only a few on-point trials, some of them poorly designed. However, they apparently had to provide an answer to the question posed by NIH. To support this universal acceptability of one cup of milk, they relied largely upon four trials that dosed lactose malabsorbers with milk products containing thirteen grams or less of lactose. These trials found no significant differences in symptom levels, compared to placebo treatments containing no lactose.

One trial from a group led by Dr. Nevin Scrimshaw at the Massachusetts Institute of Technology evaluated symptoms in lactose malabsorbing high school students after they consumed lactose-containing or lactose-free chocolate milk.[133] They received treatments in a double blind manner. Usually in such studies, subjects report symptom presence and severity during the test itself, generally on an hourly basis after consumption of the test products. However, the subjects in the Scrimshaw study did not report their symptoms until the following day. This delay, especially in teenagers, may have led to forgotten symptoms, or a time-induced blurring of differences of perception between the lactose-containing and lactose-free products. These symptoms are inherently subjective, and their recollection is prone to error. This delayed recording of symptoms is unusual for lactose intolerance studies, or carbohydrate malabsorption studies in general. This unusual methodology calls into question the validity of these results.

Another study from Cornell University subjected a group of 17 subjects to a series of six treatments of varying lactose levels in skim milk, whole milk, and water.[134] Subjects were selected based on reporting symptoms after consuming 25 g of lactose in water, but not after a water placebo. The subjects were never rigorously determined to be non-absorbers with a breath hydrogen test. During the trial, the symptoms reported after consuming 10 g of lactose in skim milk or whole milk did not differ from placebo. Here, placebo was water sweetened with saccharin. A better placebo would have been lactose-free milk, with all treatments standardized to the same level of sweetness. The gauntlet-type nature of this trial (each subject consumed six different test products over an undisclosed period), the lack of rigorous diagnosis of lactose non-absorber status, and the lack of a blinded placebo diminish the value of these results.

The third trial was not blinded with respect to lactose content of the test milk (study blinding was actually directed to varying milkfat levels) so drawing conclusions about intolerance symptoms is not appropriate.[135] A fourth trial evaluated symptoms after drinking two different amounts of milk. In the first portion of this trial, subjects showed a significant reduction in symptoms when they consumed 500 ml (about two cups) of partially lactose-free skim milk (86% lactose reduction) in comparison to drinking the same amount standard skim milk.[136] In the second portion of this trial, testing of 250 ml (about one cup) of this lactose-reduced lactose milk and regular skim milk did not show a "statistically significant" (at the standard p=<0.05 level) difference in reported symptoms between treatments; but there was a borderline significance level between treatments of 0.05-0.10. Such a statistical outcome is inconclusive for alleging no difference in symptoms between consuming lactose-containing or largely lactose-free skim milks. This research provides very weak support for the contention that no benefit was associated with the consuming the partially free lactose milk at a 250 ml (about a cup) consumption level.

In contrast to the four trials used to support the Consensus Conference conclusion, another trial casts doubt on the validity of the assertion that one cup of milk (12 grams of lactose) does not cause symptoms. A clinical study at Meharry Medical College in Nashville, TN evaluated a slightly higher level of lactose (fifteen grams).[137] A group of 45 African American high school and college students were selected from a larger group because of a positive response a breath hydrogen study, indicating malabsorption. In addition, all of these students claimed to suffer lactose intolerance symptoms after consuming a cup of milk. In the trial, they consumed either milk containing fifteen grams of lactose, or lactose-free milk. These researchers added artificial sweetener to the lactose-containing milk to match the greater sweetness of the enzyme-treated lactose-free milk. Out of 45 subjects, 30 (or 67%) reported lactose intolerance symptoms when drinking lactose-containing milk, but not when ingesting the lactose-free milk. Although these subjects ingested fifteen grams of lactose, the high prevalence of symptoms casts a long shadow on the assertion that practically all lactose intolerant individuals can consume twelve grams without symptoms. There is no physiological basis to believe that these students suffering symptoms at fifteen grams would have been free of symptoms after consuming twelve grams. This NIH Consensus Statement on the acceptability of twelve grams of lactose drew upon limited data, and ignored this obvious implication of the Meharry study.

In the real world, likely many lactose intolerant individuals can consume twelve grams of lactose without ill effect. But, there are also many who suffer significant symptoms. Like most topics in human biology, there can be huge differences among individuals in a specific trait. In summary, lactose intolerance symptoms are highly specific to the individual, and no arbitrary rule can be brought to bear to assert that any particular level of lactose-containing dairy will be acceptable to all. Furthermore, the proclivity to develop symptoms after lactose consumption will also vary with the type of milk consumed, other types of food consumed at the same time, emotional state of the individual, and likely many other factors. Each sufferer must determine his or her own tolerance to dairy. This decision cannot be based on an arbitrary rule, even when it bears the imprimatur of the NIH.

LACTOSE INTOLERANCE SEVERITY VARIES AMONG INDIVIDUALS

The results of some clinical trials and various commentaries in the literature appear to raise an existential issue about lactose intolerance, particularly at low dairy consumption levels.[138] However, the results of clinical trials cannot negate the genuine suffering that some lactose malabsorbers endure at even low levels of lactose. Part of this discrepancy may lie in the differences between the subjects recruited for these trials and the community of bona fide sufferers of lactose intolerance. The clinical trials just described generally enrolled subjects through limited advertising. Since many trials were carried out in university medical centers, they likely drew largely from employees and students for enrollees. The individuals responding to bulletin board advertisements to earn a few extra dollars may be far different from severe sufferers of lactose intolerance. Individuals with minor symptoms may have enrolled. In contrast, individuals with a history of suffering from severe symptoms may have avoided enrolling, as they did not want to subject themselves to an extremely unpleasant experience, particularly in their school or work environment.

In addition, a handful of researchers have conducted many of the studies that fail to demonstrate lactose intolerance after lactose or milk ingestion. Some of these researchers have spent decades downplaying the existence or severity of lactose intolerance. Often they have accepted funding from organizations such as the National Dairy Council that promote dairy consumption. This field would be greatly advanced by new large-scale trials conducted by objective researchers not hobbled by entrenched positions.

It bears repeating again that the failure to show symptoms of lactose intolerance in some clinical trials is in strong conflict with the numerous individuals who suffer symptoms after dairy consumption. Results of these trials cannot be used to deny or nullify the experiences of those individuals.

CLAIMED LACK OF SYMPTOMS OR ADVERSE EFFECTS IN LACTOSE MALABSORBERS APPEARS AT ODDS WITH GENETICS AND EVOLUTION

Chapter 4 detailed the strong natural selection for adult lactase persistence in dairy consuming populations, as evidenced by its rapid emergence at high frequencies in diverse populations of Africa, Asia, and Europe. This strong benefit of lactase in later childhood and adulthood suggests that lactose posed some hazard to these early dairy consumers. We do not know exactly the form or amount of dairy consumption in these populations. However, the strength of this natural selection is another line of evidence that lactose consumption by the lactose intolerant has strong negative effects (possibly the symptoms) that have powerfully affected human evolution. Another possibility is that undigested lactose decreases the nutritional benefit of dairy foods. This could result from a number of factors such as impaired nutrient absorption or adverse effects of colonic fermentation of lactose. The genetic learnings imply that intolerant individuals can benefit by consuming dairy but avoiding lactose intake. This can be achieved by consuming lactose-free dairy products or use of enzyme supplements.

WHY DO SOME ADULTS WITH GENETIC HYPOLACTASIA AVOID SYMPTOMS OF LACTOSE INTOLERANCE?

Published clinical trials demonstrate that a substantial portion of those with lactase nonpersistence do not suffer symptoms after dairy intake, particularly if the amount of lactose is small. Human physiology is exceedingly complex, and there is a limited understanding of why these people avoid symptoms. Potentially, a thorough understanding of this phenomenon could open new treatments for those with severe symptoms. Several factors may be involved in how some people with hypolactasia avoid symptoms.

First, as discussed in Chapter 4, changes in DNA methylation patterns during childhood appear to suppress activity of the lactase gene. However, evidence indicates that this shutdown in not totally complete, and some produce a variable amount of lactase after childhood.

Researchers at the University of Groningen in the Netherlands used a novel technique to measure the residual lactase activity in subjects with adult hypolactasia.[139] They took advantage of the tendency of certain plants, particularly corn (or maize), to selectively take up carbon-13 (C^{13}) from carbon dioxide during photosynthesis. C^{13} is a rare naturally occurring non-radioactive isotope of carbon (C^{12} is the most common isotope, and accounts for about 99% of the planet's carbon). These Dutch researchers fed cows a diet high in corn and extracted lactose from the milk, yielding lactose that was enriched in C^{13} compared to other dietary carbohydrates. Lactose malabsorbing subjects consumed a nondairy drink containing this lactose. If there were any residual lactase activity in the small intestine, it would break down a portion of the lactose, and there would be a brief spike in the blood of C^{13}-containing glucose and galactose (the component sugars of lactose). The investigators also used breath hydrogen to measure orocecal transit time (the time needed for material to pass from the mouth, through the stomach and small intestine, and reach the colon). They did this by measuring breath hydrogen levels at fifteen minute intervals after subjects drank the lactose beverage. Hydrogen levels increase rapidly after any lactose reaches the colon.

They found that, in this population with genetic hypolactasia, tolerant subjects (i.e. no symptoms) digested about 47% of the lactose consumed, based on C^{13} in carbon dioxide exhaled in air soon after lactose ingestion. In contrast, the intolerant subjects (with symptoms) digested only 34% of the lactose. Thus there appeared to be some residual lactase activity even in nonpersistent subjects, with greater levels in those who did not suffer symptoms. Not surprisingly, there was a huge variation among the subjects in the total amount of lactose digested, with values ranging from about 8% to over 80%. The tolerant group displayed delayed colonic hydrogen production, an indication of longer transit time, compared to the intolerant group. Hydrogen levels peaked at 248 minutes after lactose ingestion in the tolerant group, compared to a peak at 161 minutes in the intolerant group. The authors proposed that longer transit time allowed more contact of lactose with the small amount of lactase in the intestinal villi, resulting in greater breakdown. In summary, intestinal lactose breakdown in subjects with genetic hypolactasia appears to depend on both the level of "leakiness" of the enzyme repression, and the speed that ingested lactose passes by the intestinal villi containing the enzyme. If this repression is incomplete, and lactose has a sufficient contact time with this diminished enzyme, digestion may be sufficient to avoid symptoms.

Several studies more directly confirm low levels of intestinal lactase in people with adult hypolactasia. Evaluations of intestinal biopsy samples show a low level of lactase in the villi even in individuals with adult hypolactasia. For example, one study used two approaches to evaluate biopsy samples from a group of fourteen patients with suspected lactose intolerance.[140] The first consisted of assaying a portion of each biopsy sample for lactase activity. The second method was an immunochemical microscopy procedure. In this test, a monoclonal antibody reacting with lactase was applied to thin cross sections of the biopsy to identify the exact location of the enzyme in cells of the villus. This antibody was conjugated with a fluorescent marker, and under the microscope a spot of light marked the location of lactase. Both of these methods showed some residual lactase activity in all fourteen of these presumably lactose intolerant patients. Although this study predated the development of the genetic test for adult hypolactasia, several of the subjects were of African or Chinese origin, and based on their genetic background they had likely experienced shutdown of the lactase gene during adolescence. This suggests some low level of lactase production continuing in adulthood even in individuals lacking a SNP's for persistence.

A second British study corroborates these low levels of lactase.[141] Biopsy samples from eleven non-persistent patients were tested for lactase enzyme activity, and the researchers also microscopically examined them to determine the location of the enzyme activity. All of these individuals proved to have some level of residual lactase activity, and microscopic examination revealed a patchy distribution of enzyme in the brush border cells of the villi. This study was also performed before appearance of genetic test for lactase SNP's, but most of the non-persistent individuals were not of northern European origin, suggesting adult hypolactasia.

The existence of low levels of lactase production in individuals with adult hypolactasia has gained little appreciation by both the scientific and lay communities. Particularly since the discovery in the early 2000's of SNPs causing adult lactase production, researchers have generally viewed lactase absorption or malabsorption as a binary phenomenon. Either someone did not carry one to the SNPs and was a lactose malabsorber, or carried one of these SNPs and consequently was an absorber (assuming the absence of disease leading to secondary intolerance). The true situation is likely much more nuanced. Individuals without the SNPs still have some low and variable levels of lactase production. Some of these individuals may also have relatively low rates of GI passage (that is, long orocecal transit time). As noted previously, this may allow these individuals to consume low or even moderate amounts of lactose-rich dairy without overt symptoms of lactose intolerance.

THE POSSIBLE ROLE OF COLONIC ADAPTATION IN MITIGATING LACTOSE INTOLERANCE

In some adults with hypolactasia, residual intestinal lactase and slow orocecal transit may combine to eliminate much of the lactose in dairy before it reaches the colon. A second line of defense lies in the ability of the diverse community of colon microflora to metabolize lactose. In theory, some populations of bacteria may metabolize lactose without producing the abundant quantities of hydrogen that cause bloating, cramping, and flatulence. Similarly, rapid degradation of lactose may decrease the osmotic diarrhea caused by a high concentration of lactose in the colon. Enhancing levels of particular colon microflora has been extensively touted as a means for preventing or reducing the symptoms of lactose intolerance.[142] This section examines the data supporting this assertion.

"Colonic adaptation" is the term given to the concept that the colon bacteria can adapt to the various non-digestible materials that reach the colon after digestion of foods. This adaptation could shift the colon bacteria to a more benign state, in which adverse effects of the diet (such as lactose intolerance) are reduced. Colonic adaptation has often been proposed as an approach for avoiding the symptoms of lactose intolerance. It offers the tantalizing prospect that the individual could intentionally alter the microflora of the colon through diet changes, thus reducing GI symptoms.

This is an appealing and empowering concept for lactose intolerant individuals, and it has received much attention. Despite the appeal, few credible studies support it. There are scant rigorous scientific trials in this area, and the designs of some these make the results difficult to interpret. In particular, due to lack of proper control groups, it is difficult to determine whether symptoms actually decreased over time with the consumption of lactose-containing dairy products, or the individual just became used to the symptoms (like getting used to a low-grade pain).

APPROACHES TO COLONIC ADAPTATION

Two basic approaches have attempted to achieve colonic adaptation in the lactose intolerant. One approach is based on a theory that continued introduction of lactose (or a structurally similar carbohydrate) into the colon will result in an increase in the bacteria that are able to efficiently ferment lactose, and possibly ferment it in a manner that decreases gas production and osmotic effects. A second tactic, the "probiotic approach," is based on ingesting specific bacteria (in food or tablet form) that will reach the colon and alter the metabolism of lactose.

The first approach entails consuming slowly increasing levels of dairy products or lactose itself over a period of time, ranging from a couple of weeks to months. In theory, this increasing level of lactose entering the colon gives a selective advantage to groups of lactose fermenting bacteria, particularly the bifidobacteria and the lactobacilli. Multiple species of both of these genera normally reside in the colon, providing numerous candidates for adaptation process.

The environment partly determines the metabolism of colon bacteria. The colon is largely free of oxygen ("anaerobic"). In the presence of sufficient oxygen, bacteria would largely convert lactose into carbon dioxide and water. However, in the anaerobic colon a complex fermentation process occurs, and by-products of lactose produced by one group of bacteria are consumed by other bacteria as food sources. This fermentation cascade yields the gasses hydrogen, carbon dioxide, and sometimes methane, and short chain fatty acids (SCFA) such as acetic, propionic, butyric, and also lactic acid. When lactose is converted into these acids, the osmotic load increases about eight-fold compared to that exerted by lactose alone (recall that osmotic load affects the intestine's ability to retain water, and a high osmotic load is likely to lead to watery diarrhea). Consequently, if the SCFA are not efficiently absorbed through the colon wall, there is an increased tendency toward diarrhea in lactose maldigesters. However, these SCFA are also metabolized by the human body, particularly the mucosal tissues lining the colon. Rapid SCFA absorption and metabolism limits their accumulation in the colon.

A competitive process may exist between how rapidly SCFA are produced from lactose by colon bacteria, and how quickly SCFA are absorbed through the colon wall. If SCFA are absorbed rapidly, this will reduce the tendency toward diarrhea. If they are absorbed much more slowly than they are produced by bacteria, this increases the osmotic load and tendency to diarrhea. Possibly, this situation may set up a conspiratorial feedback loop to exacerbate diarrhea. The increased fluid in the colon could dilute the SCFA concentration, and slow absorption. Furthermore, diarrhea will speed up transit time through the colon, decreasing the time available for SCFA absorption.

Numerous scientific papers have speculated on colonic adaptation to lactose, and attributed great benefits to it. These publications reflects a strong desire to believe, but unfortunately robust data do not support this belief. Instead, only scant evidence supports the colonic adaptation hypothesis.

Two persuasive human trials have provided some credibility. In 1996 Drs. Stephen Hertzler and Dennis Savaiano at Purdue University conducted a 22 day trial in lactose maldigesting adults (diagnosed on the basis of a >20 ppm rise in breath hydrogen during a lactose challenge).[143] They hypothesized that colonic adaptation would be manifested by a decrease in both breath hydrogen levels and symptoms after a period of lactose consumption. In this crossover design trial, a group of 20 subjects consumed lactose or glucose for days 1-10, and then consumed the other treatment for days 12 through 21. The initial level of each sugar was 0.6g/kg of body weight per day (about 42 g for a healthy weight adult). Sugars levels were gradually increased, and the final intake level was one g/kg per day. They divided each day's sugar dose into three portions, and subjects consumed one portion in water with each meal. They performed lactose challenge tests on days 11 and 22 (thus each subject participated in a lactose challenge immediately after the dosing periods of both lactose and glucose). Notably, study results did not show a decrease in symptoms in the lactose challenge test after consuming lactose on a daily basis. As noted previously, symptom severity is difficult to measure accurately. However, breath hydrogen levels were much lower after ten days of lactose intake, compared to ten days of glucose intake. This suggests that prolonged lactose intake altered the colon microflora in some manner to decrease hydrogen production, although this did not result in a significant decrease in symptoms. One criticism of this study is that there was not a washout period (that is, a period of no treatment between the lactose and glucose consumption). If, in the group that received lactose first, it had produced a shift toward more benign lactose-metabolizing bacteria, this adaptation could have persisted through the glucose treatment period in the subjects who had consumed lactose first, possibly affecting the subsequent breath hydrogen test results. It must be noted that this study was funded by the National Dairy Board (now known as the National Dairy Promotion and Research Board), a government-created agency that promotes dairy consumption.

In a later study, Dr. Jean Claude Rambaud and his research team at the Hôpital Saint-Lazare in Paris designed a trial to determine whether the reported reduction in lactose symptoms after continued ingestion of lactose or dairy was really the result of purported colonic adaptation.[144] This experiment enrolled 46 intolerant subjects of Asian ancestry. These subjects underwent lactose (50 g) breath hydrogen challenges on the first and fifteenth days of the trial. On the days between these tests, one-half of the subjects consumed 17 g of lactose in water twice daily and other half similarly consumed sucrose. Aspartame in the sugar solutions masked the difference in sweetness between sucrose and lactose. The treatment was double-blinded, so that neither the subjects nor the researchers knew the treatment that each individual received. Importantly, this study used two groups that received treatments in parallel. Unlike the earlier cited study from Purdue, there was no crossover between treatments and hence no possibility of a persistent effect of colonic adaptation.

This French group found that breath hydrogen decreased by 55% over two weeks in the group that received the lactose solution, indicating some colonic adaptation had occurred. A 50% increase in lactase levels in stool samples from these subjects further supported beneficial changes in colon flora (fecal lactase is produced by colon bacteria). In contrast, no decrease in breath hydrogen or increase in fecal lactase occurred between beginning and end of treatment in the subjects drinking sucrose. Perplexingly, symptom scores decreased for the lactose and sucrose groups by almost identical amounts. Since no colonic adaptation to lactose could have occurred in the sucrose group, the apparent decrease in their symptom severity during their final lactose challenge could have been due to the subjects becoming accustomed to the symptoms caused by the lactose challenge (the second challenge was only two weeks after the first). Consequently, they may have become more conservative in the scores they assigned to symptoms in the second test. Regardless, the similar decrease in symptoms following both lactose and sucrose ingestion indicates that this symptom reduction was likely an artifact of the test procedure, and not entirely ascribable to colonic adaptation. That said, the observed 55% reduction in breath hydrogen in the lactose-treated subjects should plausibly have yielded an improvement in symptoms.

These two studies differ in design, but there are similarities in the results. Hertzler used a high level of lactose during the adaptation phase. The dosing of one g per kg of body weight meant that the average adult was consuming daily the amount of lactose in one-half gallon of milk. Breath hydrogen levels did decrease after ten days of lactose consumption, but not with glucose. There was no significant improvement in symptoms despite this decrease. During the treatment phase the Rambaud study used a lower daily level of lactose, similar to a quart of milk. Even at this lower treatment level hydrogen levels in a lactose challenge decreased by more than one-half over a fifteen-day treatment. However, again this decrease was not accompanied by an amelioration of symptoms ascribable to the treatment.

The lack of symptom reduction in both studies is troubling. Breath hydrogen measurements are a simple, quantitative approach for evaluating carbohydrate fermentation. Indeed, as noted previously similar tests are used to evaluate a number of carbohydrate digestion disorders. Despite widespread use, breath hydrogen levels do not appear to be strongly associated with intensity of lactose intolerance symptoms. Perhaps there is a physiological basis for this, or maybe the inherently qualitative nature of measuring symptom intensity with subject-completed numeric scales is just too imprecise to yield meaningful data. In addition, as is the case with many clinical trials on lactose intolerance, self-selection of the subjects may have compromised these studies. Individuals who knew they were likely to suffer serious symptoms at the proposed levels of lactose consumption may have declined to participate, whereas prospective subjects who expected mild symptoms may have been more willing to participate in the study. Subjects with generally mild symptoms may not have experienced a measurable reduction in symptoms because of colonic adaptation.

For the individual attempting to manage lactose intolerance, there is limited support for pursuing the colonic adaptation approach. That said, this approach is plausible and worthy of a try, as the only downside appears be enduring symptoms during the attempted colonic adaptation. As noted before, human biology is amazingly variable and some individuals may benefit greatly from attempting to acclimate to lactose with repeated consumption of dairy. Of course, for some individuals these symptoms may prove to be too severe to make this approach endurable.

POSSIBLE ROLE OF PROBIOTICS IN MITIGATING LACTOSE INTOLERANCE

Probiotics are microorganisms believed to support health, with the GI tract the most common focus. Bacteria of the genera *Lactobacillus* and *Bifidobacterium* are the most common probiotics and they are both enthusiastic metabolizers of lactose. Given this fact, and the assumption that probiotics will survive and even proliferate in the human intestine, a widespread speculation has developed that probiotics should be effective in dealing with lactose intolerance. Unfortunately, most human studies have failed to show such a benefit for probiotic supplements. The few that have shown a benefit were limited in size and sometimes flawed, and certainly need replication before probiotics can be recommended for this purpose. Please note that yogurt, which contains similar bacteria, presents quite a different story from probiotic supplements. A separate section examines the utility of yogurt.

Before delving into this possible benefit of probiotics, more background on the microbiology of the colon is warranted. Undigested food remnants reaching the colon become the growth medium for a vast assemblage of bacteria. As discussed previously, the metabolism of these bacteria make the colon a very anaerobic environment, and fermentation reactions drive metabolism. The fermentation products from one group of bacteria often become substrates for additional fermentation by other bacteria. A slightly different consortium of bacteria likely breaks down each substrate in undigested food. The immense diversity of bacteria in the colon aids this process; well over 1000 species of organisms are found in the colon.[145] The profile of colon bacteria is unique to each individual, like a fingerprint, and represents a lifelong process of adaptation by the bacteria to their unique human host. In essence, the repertoire of bacteria evolves to accommodate the unique diet and physiology of each individual. The immense diversity of bacteria present is coupled with their enormous numbers. Each gram of human feces contains up to about 10^{12} bacteria (this number, in non-exponential form, is 1,000,000,000,000 or one trillion).[146] Bacteria comprise up to 60% of the weight of human feces. Since several hundred grams or more of colon contents may be present in an individual, the total number of colon bacteria is truly immense. The number of colon bacteria vastly exceeds the number of human cells in the body.

With this background, the challenges for a probiotic supplement to alter the landscape of the colon appear substantial. A typical probiotic supplement contains about 10^8 to 10^9 bacteria (100,000,000 to 1,000,000,000). This is about as many bacteria as are present in 0.1 to 1 of mg of human fecal matter (an amount that borders on being so small as to be invisible). For a probiotic strain to establish itself as a prominent member of the colon flora, it would have to possess a powerful selective advantage.

Perhaps the probiotic does not have to overcome this challenge of numbers in the colon to provide a benefit for lactose metabolism. In most people the small intestine contains few bacteria, and many of these are transient organisms associated with food. Possibly the probiotic bacteria establishes a transient or permanent residence in the less crowded environment of the small intestine. From this location, they could produce lactase, with the sugars cleaved from lactose metabolized by these bacteria or absorbed by the host. This would limit the amount of lactose reaching the colon. This possibility is a mere hypothesis. If probiotics do have an effect on lactose intolerance, the specific site of this action is unknown.

A further issue complicating the evaluation of probiotics for lactose intolerance is the considerable number of probiotic strains that have been evaluated for this potential benefit. Each strain is physiologically different, and may differ in traits such as the ability to survive exposure to stomach acid and bile acids in the small intestine or to attach to the gut epithelium. Therefore, it is not valid to extrapolate results obtained for any particular strain of probiotics to other strains.

Another difficulty is that probiotic manufacturers have funded many of the clinical trials. Even if the manufacturers are not hands-on involved in performing a trial (that is hopefully the case) there is always the potential for publication bias. That is, if the results of the trial are favorable, publication is likely, but if the results are negative, they may just gather dust in a file drawer. Published trials in this area tend to be small, which is not surprising since many probiotics manufacturers are small companies with limited resources. Unfortunately, large scale funding from unbiased sources has generally not been available for probiotic research.

Some studies have shown a benefit for specific probiotic strains in improving lactose digestion. An Italian trial compared the effects of *Lactobacillus reuteri*, a well-studied probiotic, and a lactase enzyme tablet on breath hydrogen levels.[147] Before treatment, all subjects received a breath hydrogen test, with a 25 g lactose challenge. The study participants receiving the probiotic consumed four tablets of *L. reuteri* daily for ten days prior to breath hydrogen measurements during a lactose challenge test. A separate group consumed lactase tablets a single time, just before a second lactose challenge. When compared to results of a breath hydrogen test performed at baseline (before any treatments were consumed), subjects who had consumed the probiotic for ten days experienced an average 33% decrease in hydrogen levels, compared to a 55% reduction for subjects who consumed the lactase tablets just once. Therefore, the lactase tablets were far superior to the probiotic, even though consumed just once, in contrast to ten days of probiotic dosing. The lactase treatment group was accompanied by a placebo control (these subjects received placebo tablets, instead of lactase, just before the breath hydrogen test). However, unfortunately there was no control group for the *L. reuteri* treatment. This would have added more credibility to the probiotic results.

A small eleven-subject study in China evaluated effects of a treatment with multiple probiotics on lactose intolerance.[148] For ten days volunteers consumed a yogurt supplemented with *Bifidobacterium animalis* along with capsules containing *Bifidobacterium longum*. Researchers performed lactose challenge assays before and after this supplementation period. There was a significant decrease in symptoms after supplementation. However, the study design casts doubt on the results. There was no placebo group, and all subjects apparently knew that they were receiving a treatment intended to reduce the severity of their previously diagnosed lactose intolerance symptoms. A desire for the treatment to work, or an eagerness to please the investigators, may have swayed the subjects reported outcomes. Studies with similarly flawed designs are unfortunately quite common in the probiotic scientific literature.

A Brazilian trial compared the efficacies of a probiotic product and a lactase supplement.[149] Lactose breath hydrogen tests were used to identify malabsorbing individuals among patients attending university gastroenterology clinics. A group of 27 of these patients was subjected to two sequential treatments. The first was ingestion of lactase (two tablets of Lactaid® Extra-Strength) followed immediately by a breath hydrogen test. This test had been preceded by a breath hydrogen test that evaluated placebo tablets. The second treatment involved ingestion of Yakult probiotic powder (*Lactobacillus casei* Shirota and *Bifidobacterium breve* Yakult) mixed into water with each meal for four weeks. Patients received another breath hydrogen study at the end of four weeks. The single dose lactase treatment produced a 54% reduction in breath hydrogen, compared to only a 16% reduction after 28 days of Yakult probiotic treatment. They reported similar reductions in symptom severity for both treatments. Three months after treatment ended, the Brazilian researchers again asked the subjects to report their lactose intolerance symptoms. Overall, the probiotic group reported a continued reduction in their symptoms. However, this study lacked a parallel placebo group, which undermines validity of the patient symptom scores. The patients knew they had received treatments intended to reduce symptoms, and this could have colored their responses.

The authors of a review of probiotic clinical trials for lactose intolerance concluded that probiotics in general are not effective. [150] However, they determined that the available information suggests that some individuals respond positively to particular strains, and it is reasonable for the lactose intolerant to experiment with some of the available strains. The authors of this review summarized the situation concisely: "Probiotic supplementation in general did not alleviate the symptoms and signs of lactose intolerance in adults . . . Some evidence suggests that specific strains, concentrations, and preparations are effective. Further clinical trials of specific strains and concentrations are necessary to delineate this potential therapeutic relationship."

YOGURT

Yogurt is made by culturing milk with bacteria, and part of its characteristic taste derives from the action of these bacteria on lactose. Yogurt bacteria are typically strains of *Lactobacillus bulgaricus* and *Streptococcus thermophilus*. These organisms transport lactose into the cell, where the activity of lactase produces glucose and galactose. These bacteria then ferment these simple sugars to obtain energy, with lactic acid as the main end product that is dumped back into the milk. Lactic acid increases the acidity of the milk (to a pH of about 4.0-4.5), and provides the pungent taste of yogurt. Acidity also causes coagulation of some of the milk proteins, resulting in the semi-solid state of most yogurts. Lactase is generally located inside the bacteria, but some may leak into the environment if they are dead or damaged.

Lactose-intolerant individuals generally handle yogurt far better than they do milk. Part of the improvement is simply due to the decreased level of lactose in yogurt, compared to milk. The culturing process for yogurt typically removes about one-fourth of the lactose in the starting milk. However, some yogurt making processes involve adding milk solids, which may increase the initial lactose levels above that of milk. In addition to attacking lactose during yogurt manufacturing, these cultures may continue to break down lactose remaining in yogurt during its passage through the GI tract. A crucial factor for successful digestion of the remaining lactose in yogurt is the presence of viable bacteria. Bacteria are separated from their environment by a complex cell wall structure. The lactase enzyme is located inside the bacterial cell, and another enzyme system (lactose permease) is needed to bring lactose inside the cell where it can be broken down and converted to lactic acid. This permease system is only effective in living bacteria. Dr. Salwa Rizkalla and colleagues at the Hôtel-Dieu Hospital in Paris confirmed this need for living bacteria in a human study involving ingestion of yogurt with live cultures, or the same yogurt pasteurized to kill the bacteria. Lactose-intolerant people had much higher levels of breath hydrogen after consuming the pasteurized yogurt, compared to the unheated material.[151]

Other research supports the necessity of viable yogurt cultures for treating lactose intolerance. The specific cultures used to make the yogurt have little impact on the efficacy of the yogurt in metabolizing lactose. Dr. Dennis Savaiano and his research group at Purdue used four different yogurt cultures to prepare yogurts from whole milk.[152] He fed these yogurts (or a whole milk control) to intolerant volunteers. He then compared hydrogen production after consumption of these yogurts with hydrogen production after an equivalent amount of whole milk. Overall, hydrogen levels after yogurt consumption were only about one-third o of that from whole milk consumption, with no significant differences among the test yogurts.

Many or most lactose intolerant people should be able to enjoy yogurt with minimal or no symptoms. A few caveats are warranted. Some yogurts are pasteurized to extend their shelf life, so that they can be shipped across the continent or stored in warehouses for long periods. Consumers should obviously avoid such pasteurized products, and the yogurt label should indicate it contains live cultures. Additionally, the viability of the yogurt bacteria will decline during storage. Yogurt should be consumed before its "use by" date, and for best efficacy yogurt should be consumed quickly after purchase.

An earlier chapter reviewed the ways that early man exploited the nutritional bonanza resulting from the domestication of cattle and other milk-producers. Aside from the fortuitous appearance of adult lactase persistence, the other routes to consuming dairy without ill effect involved early dairy technology, including yogurt production. However, early yogurt probably differed greatly from what we currently purchase from supermarkets. The bacterial cultures now used in making modern industrial-scale yogurt may be vastly different from the wild strains that early pastoralists used intentionally or accidentally. These ancient bacteria were newly derived from natural sources, and likely retained the properties that allowed them to survive in difficult environments. In contrast, modern yogurt cultures have been selected (and evolved) to be highly efficient, rapid producers of mild-tasting yogurt under carefully controlled factory conditions. After decades or centuries of this environment, they may have lost the no longer needed traits for surviving hostile conditions such as the human GI tract. Thus one can reasonably speculate that the yogurts of the early pastoralists were more effective in both ameliorating the effects of lactose, and providing a broader GI benefit.

Although the lactose intolerant may find lactose in yogurt to be more digestible, it is unclear if any of this benefit transfers to consumption of other dairy products. Perhaps there is a benefit for other dairy products consumed simultaneously with yogurt, but there is no persuasive evidence that the yogurt provides a longer-lasting benefit (such as colonic adaptation).

Additionally, the benefits of yogurt are apparently not shared by other dairy products that are merely supplemented with bacteria (in contrast to yogurt, in which the bacteria introduced via a starter culture proliferate to vast numbers). Sweet acidophilus milk is prepared by adding *Lactobacillus acidophilus* bacteria to milk, but the milk is not held under conditions that permit the bacteria to proliferate and partially convert lactose to lactic acid. The milk is "sweet" because it lacks the tartness imparted by lactic acid. A study utilizing lactose intolerant volunteers compared breath hydrogen production after consumption of whole milk, sweet acidophilus milk prepared with this milk, and yogurt prepared from the whole the milk. Breath hydrogen levels were markedly reduced after consumption of the yogurt, but the sweet acidophilus milk produced no reduction in breath hydrogen in comparison to the control whole milk. The lack of effect of the sweet acidophilus milk may result simply from the decreased number of bacteria present, as compared to yogurt. On a weight basis, the sweet acidophilus milk contained only about 10-25% of the numbers of bacteria in yogurts that have been found to effectively decrease breath hydrogen levels.[153]

Yogurt appears to be an acceptable route for dairy consumption for most lactose intolerant individuals. As with other treatments, each person needs cautious experimentation to determine the effectiveness of this approach.

SUMMARY

The lactose intolerant person attempting to manage this condition without total dairy avoidance faces a range of options with varying degrees of scientific grounding. A "one cup" rule posits that the lactose intolerant can consume a cup of milk without adverse effects. This theory has been widely spread in both the lay press and the nutrition literature. However, the supporting evidence is limited. Likely some individuals can consume a cup of milk without ill effect (at least most of the time), but others may suffer uncomfortable symptoms. The variability in human biology must never be ignored.

In the absence of adult lactase production (the normal state for 70-80% of the world population), other physiological factors permit some people to consume lactose-containing dairy without ill effect. We have a poor understanding of these factors, which likely include some residual levels of lactase expression, slow intestinal motility, and the types of bacteria residing in the GI tract. Many clinical trials have attempted to alter these bacteria ("colonic adaptation") to reduce intolerance symptoms, but the overall results in this area are not persuasive. This is an area where a sufferer can reasonably experiment, though a benefit should not be assumed.

Many have touted prebiotics as a solution for intolerance, but here the scientific support is also limited. Again, experimentation by the sufferer may be warranted. Yogurt presents a markedly different situation. It possesses the benefits of both lactose content reduction during manufacturing and the residual effects of bacterial lactase after consumption.

The lactose intolerant consumer has a number of options. One effective approach not covered in this chapter is the use of lactase supplements or lactase-free dairy products. This is a rich subject area, and its development is strongly tied to the identification of lactose intolerance as a medical condition. This story unfolds in the next chapter.

11 A HISTORY OF THE DISCOVERY OF LACTOSE INTOLERANCE, AND ITS TREATMENT

The previous chapters explored the origins of human dairy cultures, and the genetic changes that led to a world with a divide between adult lactase producers (persistent), and non-producers (non-persistent). Some of the non-persistent are able to consume certain amounts of dairy without developing extensive symptoms of lactose intolerance. Other non-persistent individuals undeniably do suffer major symptoms after consuming lactose-containing dairy products. Earlier chapters briefly noted some of the treatments available to these persons. This chapter will delve more deeply into these treatments, and summarize the science supporting their efficacy (or sometimes lack of efficacy).

RECOGNITION OF LACTOSE TOLERANCE AND INTOLERANCE IS RELATIVELY RECENT

Beginning with the history of the recognition of lactose intolerance as a health issue is appropriate. Effective treatments were only developed after the symptoms and their cause were understood, and human ingenuity could be brought to bear on solving the newly defined problem. The history of the science in this area and the development of treatments are inexorably intertwined.

A general understanding of the human digestive process emerged in the 18th and 19th centuries. Scientists had determined that acid and proteases in the stomach initiated the digestive process. They also found that the pancreas produces several other digestive enzymes (proteases, amylase, and lipase) and secretes these along with bile into the small intestine. These enzymes help to complete the digestive process. The early view was that enzymes from the pancreas largely carried out digestion in the intestinal lumen.[154]

Lactase is present in the intestinal epithelium, and it acts in situ (rather than secreted into the lumen of the intestine, as are the pancreatic enzymes). The understanding of the key digestive roles of lactase and other enzymes attached to the intestinal epithelium developed more slowly, but by the late 19th century the recognition of lactose as the sugar in milk and the role of lactase in its digestion were well established. Physiologists identified the presence of lactase in the intestinal epithelium of young mammals in the 1890's, as well as its loss as the animals became adults.[155] However, there were conflicting reports on whether the consumption of lactose or milk by adult animals could restore production of the enzyme. Lab assays for lactase activity at that time were inaccurate and time-consuming, and this likely contributed to the confusing literature. For decades after these early investigations, there seems to have been an implicit assumption in the scientific literature that humans differed from other mammals in maintaining lactase production into adulthood. During the later 19th century, most scientific research was conducted in Europe (primarily northern Europe) and the United States. It was likely done by mostly lactase-persistent investigators of northern European ancestry. The view at that time that all adult humans were lactase producers perhaps derived from an unconscious cultural narrow-mindedness. Regardless, there appears to have been an assumption for several decades that adult lactase persistence was the "normal" human condition.

Work led by Arne Dalqvist at the University of Lund in Sweden decisively overturned this assumption in 1963.[156] Dr. Dalqvist had been investigating the enzymes in the intestinal epithelium. To aid his work, he developed an accurate, sensitive method for measuring lactase and other digestive enzymes in the tiny samples of tissue obtained from intestinal biopsies.[157] As is often the case in science, the development of new tools empowered discoveries that overthrew widely held beliefs. His work on developing enzymes assays for these tiny tissue samples set the stage for the rapid advancement of knowledge about human lactase. While working in Chicago, Dahlqvist and other researchers identified four male patients who developed discomfort and diarrhea after drinking milk. In tests in the clinic, they consumed solutions of lactose, and he measured their blood glucose levels. The blood glucose curves were flat, indicating an absence of functional levels of lactase. Dahlqvist assayed the levels of three carbohydrate digesting enzymes (sucrase, isomaltase, and lactase) in duodenal biopsies from these men, as well as in similar biopsies from three men who could digest lactose, as evidenced by a rise in glucose after drinking milk. These three controls had normal levels of all three enzymes. In contrast, the lactose intolerant men had normal levels of two enzymes, but their lactase levels were only about 6% of the control levels. This work for the first time tied together lactose intolerance symptoms and the absence of effective levels of intestinal lactase. It clearly demonstrated that lactose intolerance resulted from the deficiency in a specific enzyme, and (at least in these subjects) it was not the result of a larger disruption of the intestinal surface since the other enzymes were present in normal levels. This pivotal research led to an outpouring of studies by other researchers in the 1960's that began to reveal the ethnic differences in lactase production. This torrent of research has continued for the last half century.

The work by Dahlqvist and similar studies demonstrated that many adult humans lack effective levels of lactase. However, a false presumption held by many scientists slowed further progress in unraveling this area. In 1953 James Watson and Francis Crick (and other, less recognized collaborators) showed that the double helix structure of DNA was the mechanism responsible for carrying genetic information. However, for some time after this there was little understanding of how cells actually converted this information into proteins that enabled them to cope with changing conditions. Investigations in bacteria helped to solve this riddle. In 1961 Francois Jacob and Jacques Monod, two French scientists, showed that lactase in *E. coli*, the common gut bacterium, was inducible. This means that the bacteria do not normally produce lactase in the absence of lactose. However, when exposed to lactose as the sole energy source, the bacteria produce copious amounts of lactase. In the absence of lactose, a repressor protein binds to the DNA promoter region that controls lactase production. If lactose is present in the environment, some diffuses into the cell. Lactose attaches to the repressor, triggering its release from the chromosome. This allows the transcription of messenger RNA for lactase, which quickly leads to the production of large amounts of lactase. The bacteria can then utilize this new energy source. Jacob and Monod received the Nobel Prize in Physiology or Medicine in 1965 for their discovery, which was monumentally pivotal to the progress of molecular biology. This discovery mesmerized the biologists of that time. Scientists extrapolated the relatively simple Jacob-Monod model of enzyme induction in bacteria to explain the production of many human enzymes, including lactase. The available facts seemed to support a related theory: populations with continuous exposure to dairy generally had effective levels of intestinal lactase, whereas dairy non-consumers lacked lactase. Again, by analogy with the *E. coli* discovery, many scientists believed that if non-lactase producing humans continually ingested dairy, this would induce lactase production in their intestines, and they would become lactose intolerant. Today, we know that very few human enzymes are inducible via the process discovered by Jacob and Monod, and human lactase is certainly not inducible. However, this erroneous extrapolation of bacterial lactase genetics to humans colored the literature on lactose intolerance for some time, with frequent suggestions (or commands) that dairy consumption would induce lactase, leading to lactose tolerance. This viewpoint perhaps slowed the development of the field, until new research put science back on the tracks.

UNDERSTANDING THE ETHNIC DIFFERENCES IN LACTASE PERSISTENCE

Dr. Pedro Cuatrecasas and colleagues at Johns Hopkins University reported in early 1965 that adult lactose malabsorption was more common in black residents of Baltimore, compared to a similar group of whites.[158] However, they recognized that the black group was composed of largely non-milk drinkers, and, in line with the current belief, attributed the absence of lactase to the absence of enzyme induction that would accompany milk consumption.

Separately, a young gastroenterologist, Dr. Theodore Bayless, became interested in lactose intolerance while serving as an Army Captain at the Tropical Research Laboratory in San Juan, Puerto Rico. He was studying tropical sprue, an intestinal disease characterized by chronic diarrhea, weight loss, and malabsorption. He noticed that many of his patients complained of diarrhea caused by the milk that they were served with each meal. Using the disaccharidase assay obtained from Arne Dahlqvist, he found that biopsy samples taken from patients with active sprue had diminished levels of sucrase, isomaltase, and lactase. After antibiotic treatment for sprue, isomaltase and sucrase activity quickly recovered. However, about a year passed before lactase levels returned to normal. This sparked his continuing interest in lactose malabsorption. He began to suspect ethnic differences in adult lactase activity after he separately tested biopsies from four black men, and found them all to be low in lactase.

After joining the faculty at Johns Hopkins, he conducted a larger study to verify ethnic differences in adult lactase persistence.[159] He and colleagues studied a group of 40 volunteers, consisting of 20 blacks and 20 whites. They found that 15 of the blacks had a flat blood glucose curve after lactose challenge (indicative of low intestinal lactase). In contrast, only two whites had flat glucose curves. Similarly, 14 of the blacks had biopsy lactase levels of less than two units, whereas only one white had such low lactase. These authors attributed adult lactose malabsorption in blacks to genetic selection in Africa that minimized the persistence of lactase in adults. Trypanosomiasis, a disease spread by the tsetse fly, prevents cattle raising in much of tropical Africa. The authors speculated that the lack of milk availability after infancy was a selective factor against the persistence of lactase in adulthood. This publication triggered a prescient letter to the authors by a Nigerian doctor (Dr. B. Ransome-Kuti). He explained that the authors "had it all wrong, that low levels of lactase after weaning was the norm and that whites had a lactase excess."[160]

In early 1968, Drs. Bayless and Shi-Shung Huang reported in the prestigious journal Science that 19 of 20 individuals with East Asian backgrounds (China, Philippines) were lactose intolerant.[161] This finding, in combination with their earlier report that most adult blacks in Baltimore were lactase deficient, led them to conclude "the bulk of world's population is probably intolerant to milk." This view is widely accepted today, but in 1968 it was a quite noteworthy finding. Dr. Bayless, in a long series of further studies, contributed greatly to the present understanding of the differences in adult lactase persistence in various populations. Concurrent with the publications cited here, numerous reports began to appear from far-flung parts of the globe on the frequency of lactose absorption and malabsorption in local populations. Scientists quickly documented the extent of this condition in much of the world's population, and tables began to appear detailing the extent of lactase persistence in diverse worldwide populations.

On a clinical level Dr. Bayless and colleagues recognized that, particularly in non-white patients, many complaints of recurrent abdominal pain could be due to lactase non-persistence, and elimination dairy foods could resolve the symptoms.[162] Although the consequences of adult lactase non-persistence was gaining attention at this time, Dr. Bayless was a pioneer in associating this physiological effect with the GI issues reported by many minority patients in the clinic. This work firmly established in the medical literature that lactase non-persistence and lactose malabsorption caused persistent GI issues in a large segment of the population.

Given the nutritional value of dairy products, the increasing admonitions by Dr. Bayless and other medical professionals for sensitive individuals to avoid dairy likely stimulated human creativity to devise dairy products without lactose (and created a new marketing opportunity for such products). This topic will be considered shortly. First we will explore how the recognition of widespread lactose malabsorption drove shifts in global nutrition policy.

INFLUENCE OF THE UNDERSTANDING OF LACTOSE INTOLERANCE ON FOREIGN AID POLICY

In the 1960's and 70's, developed countries frequently provided food aid to Africa, Latin America, and Asia, where many children suffered from malnutrition. In the United States, the US Agency for International Development (USAID) ran the Food for Peace program, though the Department of Agriculture played a strong role in providing commodities and nutritional guidance for the program. These food aid programs often focused on distribution of surplus food commodities, and in the US powdered milk was a major excess commodity from the dairy industry. Childhood development was a prime focus of these programs, and USAID distributed food aid to school meals and to mothers of young children. The recognition that lactose malabsorption was common in the school age children of these regions led to concerns that lactose in powdered milk could cause GI upsets. According to Drs. Bayless and Huang, reports of stomach pains in children consuming reconstituted milk substantiated this concern, though others made erroneous attempts to blame the symptoms on unsanitary conditions used to prepare milk from the powder. Because of these stomach upsets, users in some locations blended powdered milk with other foods to reduce the lactose content. Anecdotal reports indicated that milk powder was so lowly regarded that it ended up in whitewash used to paint walls. A study in undernourished Australian Aboriginal children indicated that lactose-containing milk was less nutritious (as measured by weight gain) than similar lactase-treated milk containing only 18% of normal lactose levels. In-hospital weight gain by children consuming the lactose-reduced milk was 70% greater than for children receiving the milk with the normal level of lactose. In these children, all of whom were under three years of age, lactose malabsorption was apparently due to their poor nutritional status (secondary lactose malabsorption). The authors concluded "our findings should re-emphasize the global implications of aid programmes which use milk produced by a basically lactose-tolerant Western world."[163] Overall, the controversy over providing lactose-containing milk to school age malabsorbing children appears to be still unresolved, from either a policy or scientific standpoint. Perhaps this is the result of vested interests firmly enmeshed in their viewpoints. One common argument has been that symptoms could be largely avoided if lactose-containing milk were gradually introduced into the diet (as noted in an earlier chapter, this is a recurrent belief in the literature that is not backed up by strong evidence). A supporting commentary in the Journal of American Dietetic Association stated "provided milk is introduced into the diet gradually, there are no significant difficulties attending the consumption of these supplementary amounts of skim milk." However, the commentator admittedly based this statement on "general observations", and acknowledged "definitive studies have not been made." Science is based on well-controlled studies, and conclusions based on unverifiable "general observations" lack credibility.[164]

Long after lactose malabsorption gained widespread public recognition, the USAID seemed to maintain a willful ignorance of this issue, and continued to target large amounts of powdered milk to mainly lactose-malabsorbing children in Africa and Latin America. Even in 1988, the Food for Peace Office's *Commodities Reference Manual* was silent about lactose malabsorption, merely stating "NFDM (nonfat dry milk) should be used with caution in age groups or areas not accustomed to drinking milk."[165] The overall motives for the Food for Peace program were not always so noble, and "Food for War" was perhaps a more appropriate name in some situations, as some governments sold food aid to raise funds to support or feed their militaries. In addition, it was used in rural pacification programs, such as the "Frijoles y Fusiles" (Beans and Rifles) campaign during the three decades long Guatemalan civil war. US food aid fed indigenous peoples who had been driven from their fields and villages and into resettlement camps where they could be closely surveilled by a suspicious government.[166]

Despite the lack of public consensus on the health consequences of lactose-malabsorbing children consuming milk, scientific recognition of this issue was one of the factors that served as an impetus for developing lactose-free high protein beverages that could be substituted for milk in international food aid programs. Dr. Virginia Holsinger, a scientist at the United States Department of Agriculture research center in the Wyndmoor neighborhood of northwest Philadelphia, developed a drink mix that combined soy flour with whey powder, a protein-rich but lactose-free byproduct of cheese production.[167] Such mixes were provided in large volumes to children in predominantly lactose-malabsorbing parts of the world in the 1970's. Coincidentally, Dr. Holsinger had a prominent role in developing technology for creating lactose-free milk, to be addressed shortly.

An obvious question is why develop a soy-containing beverage, instead of just treating the abundant surplus of dairy milk with lactase to eliminate lactose, and then drying this to yield lactose free powdered milk. Glucose, along with galactose, are simple sugars produced when lactase cleaves the disaccharide lactose. The problem lies in glucose being much more chemically reactive than lactose. In powdered milk made with lactase-treated milk, glucose reacts with some milk proteins to produce a brown color and a sharp, bitter taste. The resulting product is not palatable for humans. Similar problems occur in condensed milk made from lactase-treated milk.[168]

DAIRY INDUSTRY RESPONSES TO LACTOSE INTOLERANCE PUBLICITY

The suggestion that some people could not digest lactose (present in all the milk sold until the late 1970's) and that they should therefore avoid milk was met with resistance from some portions of the dairy industry, which tried to protect the halo of milk as healthy (and perhaps essential) for everyone. This controversy came to a head in 1974 when the Federal Trade Commission filed a complaint against the California Milk Advisory Board and its advertising agency related to a multi-year advertising campaign on the health benefits of milk. This campaign's theme was "Every body (sic) needs milk", and it delivered multimedia messages to

California consumers about the essentiality of milk for health, an alleged reduction in flu and colds resulting from milk consumption, and the underlying theme that everyone could consume milk. After five years and 18,000 pages of documents, a court found in 1979 that the advertising overall was not misleading. However, the decision did state "it was unfair and misleading . . . to represent to lactase deficient persons, who constitute a substantial segment of the population, that the consumption of a large or unlimited quantity of milk at a time is beneficial."[169] This ruling demonstrates that a scientific understanding of the prevalence of lactose intolerance, as developed in the 1960's, was followed by a general public recognition in the 1970's. As is typical when scientific information passes from the laboratory to the general media, there was considerable oversimplification and misinterpretation. However, this translation of scientific knowledge into a lay understanding of the condition created a new and unmet consumer need, setting the stage for development of products and therapies for treatment.

At the same time that scientists such as Dr. Bayless were learning about the widespread nature of lactose malabsorption, improvements in chemical processing and enzyme biotechnology were creating tools for reducing the lactose content of milk and developing lactase dietary supplements. The following story of the development of products for treating lactose intolerance is an interesting convergence of emerging food technology and medical knowledge.

DEVELOPMENT OF REDUCED LACTOSE AND LACTOSE FREE DAIRY PRODUCTS

In the early 1970's industrial enzyme companies turned their interest to developing food grade lactases. These companies already produced many food-processing enzymes from a wide range of microorganisms. These were used in diverse food applications such baking, beverage processing, and brewing. Development of commercial lactases was an obvious new business opportunity. One commercial lactase was derived from a yeast (then known as *Saccharomyces*, later to undergo a taxonomic change to *Kluyveromyces*), and another was from a filamentous fungus (*Aspergillus*). Oddly, one of the first applications of these new lactases was not for treating lactose intolerance, but rather in cheese technology. A research team led by Dr. Virginia Holsinger (developer of the previously mentioned lactose-free beverage) discovered that the ripening of Swiss cheese could be accelerated by treating milk with lactase during an early stage of the cheese-making process. (Unfortunately, the cheese also had a shorter shelf life because of texture changes after ripening, limiting the commercial benefit of this technology.)

Although companies had developed these enzymes for food processing rather than human therapeutics, their availability led to a flurry of human clinical trials evaluating them. It should be noted that at that time there were fewer constraints on human experimentation than exist now.

USE OF LACTASE TO TREAT LACTOSE MALABSORPTION

In 1966 researchers in London reported possibly the first use of the new lactases to treat lactose intolerance.[170] A one-year-old child was hospitalized with severe enteritis and accompanying secondary lactose intolerance. His doctor fed him a mixture of breast milk treated with lactase, along with infant formula. The proportion of treated breast milk in the diet was gradually increased. With this treatment, he began to gain weight and returned to normal after a few weeks. Although just one case study, this was supportive of the idea that the newly developed lactases could be safe and useful for humans.

Drs. David Paige, Theodore Bayless, and Shi-Sung Huang at Johns Hopkins published results of the first clinical trial of a lactose-reduced milk in 1975.[171] In this study, lactase non-persistent black youths in Baltimore received untreated (full lactose) milk, or milk treated with enzyme to reduce the lactose content by 50% or 90%. Consumption of both treated milks resulted in rapid increases in blood glucose compared to the untreated milk, with the 90% reduced milk showing the greatest rise. In fact, the glucose rise with the 90% reduced milk was similar to the glucose rise in a parallel group of lactase persistent youths who consumed untreated milk. This indicated that in lactose intolerant individuals, the glucose produced by the enzyme treatment of milk was absorbed in a manner similar to glucose absorption from milk lactose in lactose-tolerant individuals. The lactase non-persistent youths avoided symptoms when they consumed the treated milk. The authors recommended consumption of 90% reduced lactose milk by malabsorbers because of the observed glucose absorption. Three similar trials by other researchers over the next two years confirmed this initial report on lactose-reduced milk. These all determined that lactose-reduced milk was safe, well-tolerated, and could alleviate symptoms in non-absorbers.[172,173]

These trials established that reduced lactose milk was a safe and effective food for the lactose intolerant. Aside from the reduced lactose level, the only difference from conventional milk was a sweeter taste (glucose and galactose are sweeter than the parent lactose). However, users did not generally find this increased sweetness to be objectionable. Hence, with the appearance of commercial lactase and the confirmation of the effectiveness and acceptability of reduced lactose milk, the stage was set for low lactose milk to appear on store shelves.

At this point lactase had become commercially available, and researchers established its efficacy in reducing the lactose content of milk. This set the stage for commercialization of reduced lactose milk to satisfy an unmet consumer need. One would think that a major dairy company would have quickly brought its extensive resources to bear on this opportunity. However, as so often happens in innovation, a single determined individual upstaged major corporations.

Alan Kligerman was a middle-aged man with entrepreneurial skills and vast dairy knowledge (from hands-on experience in a family dairy established in 1918, and as a student in the dairy program at Cornell University). Working from the seashore resort region of southern New Jersey where he had grown up, he had gained expertise in marketing specialty food products. First, he developed a low sugar ice cream for diabetics (Sugar-Lo®) that achieved considerable success. Unfortunately, the US FDA banned cyclamate, the sweetener in Sugar-Lo®, in 1969, abruptly ending his business. Next, he turned his creativity to commercializing a dairy-free frozen dessert. The market for this never really developed, and Alan suffered another business setback. However, this did not suppress his quest for innovation.

At this time, he was aware of the problem of lactose intolerance (as noted earlier, knowledge from academic research on lactose intolerance gained increased public awareness in the early 1970's). He pragmatically began pulling together pieces of knowledge in this area. By a stroke of luck, he was conveniently close to two resources important in the eventual development of reduced lactose milk. He learned of the work of Drs. Bayless and Paige at Johns Hopkins University in nearby Baltimore. He met with them to understand the benefits of milk with reduced lactose levels, and the extent of lactose breakdown needed to make milk beneficial to lactose intolerance sufferers. Second, he traveled west to the USDA lab in Wyndmoor, Pennsylvania. Aided no doubt by persistence and charm, he was able to enlist enthusiastic help from the USDA researchers with lactase dairy application expertise, particularly Drs. Marvin Thompson, Virginia Holsinger, and Eugene Guy. He served a role as a messenger and translator of the medical knowledge emerging from Johns Hopkins clinical program. The USDA began working on lactose-free milk in their laboratories, and Kligerman developed a commercial scale process (versus the lab-scale work that had supplied reduced lactose milk for the earlier studies at Johns Hopkins).

A reduced lactose milk that a consumer could pluck out of the grocer's dairy case was the ideal product. However, putting a new dairy product on the market requires a considerable investment in obtaining production time in a dairy, developing packaging, and covering the cost of distribution. Fresh dairy products face an additional burden of short shelf life; most fluid milk must be purchased within about 14 days of production. Any milk not sold by then is a total loss, and its disposal incurs additional costs. For a new dairy product that is unknown to most potential users, this could mean a substantial number of cartons expiring prior to sale. Mr. Kilgerman pragmatically found a quicker route to the marketplace.

Lactaid®, the first consumer offering targeting the lactose intolerant, first appeared in 1976.[174] It was a box of packets of lactase. The user added the contents of the packet to a quart of milk, mixed it thoroughly, and returned it to the refrigerator. After about 24 hours, the enzyme reduced lactose by about 70%. Holding the milk under refrigeration for a longer period or the use of more enzyme could achieve even lower lactose levels. *Kluyveromyces* yeast was the source of this enzyme, which has an advantage of working well at refrigeration temperatures.

Consumers initially purchased Lactaid® only by mail order, but was later available in stores when the enzyme became available as an easier to use liquid. The enzyme packets had the benefits of longer shelf, and since refrigeration was not required, they could be shipped by any means and placed on any store shelf.

The enzyme packet of course was inconvenient for many consumers because the milk treatment required a full day. Prehydrolyzed milk offered greater convenience, and Kligerman continued his pursuit of this goal. The initial process for making Lactaid® milk resembled the use of drops by consumers. During a dairy's filling of milk cartons, a pump sprayed a small amount of micropore filtered (essentially sterile) lactase into each carton. Packaged milk usually takes a least a day to get from the dairy to the consumer's shopping cart, and by that time 70% of the lactose would be broken down. Kligerman first sold Lactaid® milk prepared by this process in eastern Pennsylvania in 1979. It quickly found a small but loyal consumer reception, and Kligerman obtained distribution in an increasing number of stores in the northeastern states. Over the following years, licenses with a number of dairy producers led to distribution over the entire United States. The initial Lactaid® milk featured a 70% lactose reduction. The commercialization of a 70% reduction was not based on technical grounds, but rather conformed to FDA regulations requiring at least a 70% reduction in order to use "reduced lactose" on the label. A "completely" (greater than 99%) lactose free product was later introduced. To achieve this, dairies conducted the enzyme treatment in large tanks, and then packaged the lactose-free milk into cartons. In this modified process, milk was flash pasteurized, treated for a prescribed time with lactase, and then pasteurized again. The first pasteurization reduced the bacterial content of the milk, and prevented development of off-flavors during the enzyme treatment. The second pasteurization destroyed any microorganisms introduced during the enzyme treatment. In summary, this highly stable milk left the dairy already free of lactose, and had a secondary benefit of a long shelf life arising from the second ultrapasteurization.

The lactose free dairy category is now over three decades old and remains a very substantial business. Lactaid® is among the bestselling milk brands in the US. It is curious that, during the time of rapid development of understanding of lactose intolerance in the 1960's and 1970's, large dairy companies sat on their hands and watched this opportunity pass them by. This should have been a very appealing area, since lactose free dairy offered the potential of higher profits in an industry characterized by abysmally low margins. Instead, they allowed this area to be seized by an entrepreneur with limited resources. Perhaps the large dairy companies were so committed to downplaying the significance of lactose intolerance that they could not recognize, or act on, an obvious business opportunity. Their indifference was followed by many years of antipathy by many dairy interests toward lactose-free milk; they remained reluctant to yield ground on their entrenched position that conventional dairy was good for everyone.

CURRENT REDUCED LACTOSE DAIRY PRODUCTS

Today lactose intolerant consumers in the US have access to two national brands of lactose-free milk, Lactaid® and Dairy Pure® (formerly Dairy Ease®). These claim to be "100% lactose free". However, it is unlikely that the enzyme reaction goes all the way to completion. These products probably still contain some residual levels of lactose (less than 1% of the original), certainly too low to have a physiological effect on consumers. Numerous store brands are also available. The current lactose-free dairy section blossoms with products from various manufacturers and includes all of the fluid milk products, including fat level variations and added flavors.

The lactose-free dairy category extends beyond milk. For example, in addition to fluid milk the Lactaid® brand offers lactose-free eggnog in season, several flavors of ice cream, and cottage cheese. Ice cream is a particularly beneficial offering. Dried milk solids, which contain large amounts of lactose, are often added to ice cream during manufacture. Thus on a volume basis ice cream may contain much more lactose than does milk. This effect is somewhat mitigated by the high fat content of ice cream, which slows the emptying of the stomach. The elevated lactose level may account for why some lactose intolerant people are especially sensitive to ice cream, and lactose-free ice cream is certainly a boon to these individuals who suffer after conventional ice cream.

Most lactose-free milk production still relies on treatment with lactase. However, dairy technologists have long pursued an alternative approach of removing lactose from milk by filtration processes. Such a process could eliminate the use of added enzyme, a potential cost-savings. The tendency of the proteins and fat in milk to clog the microfilters used to remove the lactose have hampered development of filtration. However, a few products have reached the marketplace. One example is Fairlife®, produced by a collaboration between the Coca-Cola® Company and a dairy group. In this process, microfiltering milk removes about 65% of the lactose. A traditional lactase treatment removes the remaining lactose, resulting in a very complicated overall process. This product is lower in sugar than standard milk, but has more protein and calcium than regular milk. However, despite decades of R&D efforts, filtration processes have largely not succeeded on a commercial basis, and lactase treatment remains the primary technology.

DEVELOPMENT OF LACTASE SUPPLEMENTS

In parallel with the development of lactose-free milk, the appearance of food grade lactase opened the door to enzyme supplements that could be swallowed or chewed by the consumer. In theory, this would allow a lactose intolerant person to consume any dairy product, and the ingested enzyme would break down lactose inside the body. Development of enzyme supplements was more difficult than the development of lactose-free milk for a number of reasons. First, measurement of effectiveness was a challenge. In producing lactose-free milk, very simple, accurate lab assays could measure the extent of lactose breakdown. In contrast, human efficacy of enzyme supplements could only be measured with the problematic assays discussed earlier such as the breath hydrogen test, blood glucose test or, most tricky of all, trying to measure the severity of intolerance symptoms.

In addition, during the 1970's and 1980's the United States Food and Drug Administration looked upon dietary supplement companies with strong disapproval, and pursued legal actions and product seizures. Regulatory uncertainty cast a cloud over this entire product category. Supplements only received official regulatory status after passage of the Dietary Supplement Health and Education Act in 1994.

Third, development of lactase supplements required formulating the enzyme, a delicate protein, into tablets without degrading the enzyme. This lactase had to remain potent inside the tablet for a reasonable amount of time, typically one to two years.

Finally, at first it was unclear whether any of the commercially available enzymes would be effective inside the human body, and how much enzyme would need to be consumed to degrade the lactose in servings of various dairy foods. The amount of lactase needed to treat a tank of milk in a dairy can be readily determined. In contrast, the human GI tract is far more complex (and hostile) to supplement enzymes, and clinical trials were needed to understand the amount of lactase that had to be consumed with a glass of milk, or a couple of scoops of ice cream.

Despite these difficulties, some lactase dietary supplements (for example, Lactrase®) began to appear in health food stores in the early 1980's. However, the earliest products were apparently not supported by any data indicating that they worked in the human body[175] (situations like this contributed to FDA's low regard for the supplement industry). Alan Kligerman, already established as the innovator of Lactaid® milk, turned his attention to the enzyme supplement opportunity. In this endeavor, he cooperated with a collaborator who had earlier conducted pediatric studies on the effects of lactose-free milk. This cooperative effort would be critical to the clinical validation of the lactase supplement.

Dr. Noel Solomons was a Harvard-trained American physician working with low income patients in Guatemala in the late 1970's. This tall young black man towered over his short-statured patients of largely Mayan descent. He dealt with the varied health needs of this impoverished population and, with little material support, had already developed a nutrition research program. By this point, he had already published a number of pioneering clinical trials on measuring breath hydrogen levels and evaluating the effects of diet on lactose intolerance. He fortuitously met Mr. Kligerman through Dr. Paige at Johns Hopkins, a mutual contact, at a scientific meeting in 1979. Building on their mutual interest in lactose intolerance, they soon embarked on a novel program to evaluate the efficacy of lactase in humans. This work provided an understanding of the in vivo efficacy of lactase. It also compared the in vivo efficacy of commercially available enzymes. Dr. Solomons methodically published results of numerous clinical trials evaluating several enzymes, exploring various routes of consumption, and comparing efficacy under a range of food intakes.

He knew that physicians had long used supplements of pancreatic enzymes to treat digestive deficiencies associated with diseases such as cystic fibrosis. However, pharmaceutical companies extracted these enzymes from the hog pancreas, and they had the intrinsic properties needed to survive and work in the human small intestine. In contrast, there was little history on the use of fungal enzymes as human digestive aids, and it was possible that acid and proteases in the stomach would quickly inactivate them. Initial work aimed to resolve this question. Solomons and colleagues first added lactases from various sources to milk immediately before ingestion by lactose malabsorbing children. Then, they evaluated the youths' breath hydrogen responses.[176] They found that the enzymes did work in vivo, but more enzyme had to be consumed along with milk to reduce breath hydrogen, compared to the amount of enzyme needed to effectively treat the same amount of milk in vitro (for example, refrigerating the mix of milk and enzyme overnight before consumption). Subsequent work demonstrated considerable differences in in vivo efficacy among the available lactases, with a preparation from the fungus *Aspergillus oryzae* showing the best activity.[177] Lactase preparations from this fungus are widely used in dietary supplements today. This demonstration that lactase worked in vivo when consumed with milk was followed by human trials confirming that enzyme activity was maintained when the milk was consumed as part of complex meal. These studies showed that the enzyme worked under the real world conditions of how most individuals consume milk or dairy products.[178] This validated the scientific and commercial potential of a lactase supplement. Subsequent studies demonstrated that lactase formulated into a tablet (Lactaid® Caplets) reduced both breath hydrogen and lactose intolerance symptoms when consumed along with milk by lactose-malabsorbing children.[179] This verified that the enzyme retained its activity when provided in a convenient form.

Lactaid® tablets were first sold in 1985. The user could chew them with the first bite (or sip) of dairy, or swallow the tablets intact. They filled a heretofore unmet consumer need, and rapidly became a national brand in the United States. Several versions of the Lactaid® supplement are sold today in the United States and Canada, and numerous generic products are available.

The widespread sale and consumption of lactose-free dairy products and lactase supplements has been largely limited to the United States and Canada. Perhaps a major factor in this is the ethnic diversity of these countries. Many countries with large dairy consumption (particularly northern Europe) have populations that are largely lactase persistent, and there is less potential demand for lactose-free products. In some other regions, most of the population is non-persistent, and (until recently) dairy products were not a significant portion of the diet. In contrast, the United States and Canada are a region with high dairy consumption and much ethnic diversity, yielding a large population who could benefit from these products. However, concerned consumers in much of world have access to lactase supplements. Japan, in particular, has a wide range of products, an indication of the "Westernization" of some of the diet.

More recently, consumption of lactose free dairy products has become more common in Europe and Latin America.[180] This is perhaps due to greater ethnic diversity (particularly in Europe) and efforts by enzyme suppliers to develop broader international markets.

Unfortunately, after Dr. Solomons' previously discussed pioneering efforts little additional research has occurred to improve the efficacy of lactase supplements. Questions such as how long the enzyme remains active in the GI tract and the relative amount of efficacy occurring in the stomach versus the small intestine are unanswered. We do know that the supplement lactases, typically obtained from two species of *Aspergillus* (*A. niger* and *A. oryzae*) are generally most effective at a pH of 4.5. pH is a measure of acidity or alkalinity; pure water has a pH of about 7, and a strong acid has a pH of about 0. The pH scale is logarithmic, and the level of acid changes tenfold with each one unit change in pH. The activity of the fungal enzyme decreases markedly as the pH increases or decreases from the optimum of 4.5. The fasting stomach has a pH of around 1, similar to dilute hydrochloric acid (the fasting stomach contents are basically a small pool of hydrochloric acid). After food consumption, the pH of the stomach contents rises due to the buffering activity of the ingested food. However, food consumption triggers the stomach lining to produce more acid, and the pH again falls to extremely acidic levels during the digestion process in the stomach. The acidic condition of the post-meal stomach is not only not optimal for activity of the lactase, but also eventually destroys the enzyme. Thus it would appear that most of the activity of ingested lactase in the stomach would occur during the brief period of diminished stomach acidity.

Passage of digested material from the stomach into the small intestine begins soon after the consumption of food begins. Any lactase that survives a bout with stomach acid and passes into the small intestine faces a very different environment. As partially digested material leaves the stomach, it mixes with bicarbonate buffer secreted by the small intestine. The small intestine contents become roughly neutral pH (7.0) or slightly alkaline. The lactase is very stable in this environment, but the pH is far above the optimal pH (4.5) for activity of the enzyme. However, the enzyme will be able to attack lactose during the lengthy passage of digesta through the small intestine before eventually reaching the colon (generally about 90 to 120 minutes).

One clever experiment at the University of Nagoya in Japan did explore the activity of lactase in the stomach.[181] In this study, volunteers were fitted with nasogastric tubes that permitted sampling of the stomach contents. This work used

Aspergillus oryzae lactase provided by Amano Enzyme Co. (a major producer of supplement enzyme). Volunteers ingested the enzyme under two sets of conditions: (1) enzyme ingested 30 minutes before drinking 300 ml (around 12 ounces) of skim milk containing about 18 grams of lactose, and (2) enzyme ingested simultaneously with drinking the same amount of skim milk. The researchers extracted samples of the gastric contents at the time of milk consumption, and every fifteen minutes for the following hour. They tested the samples for pH and lactase activity. When the subjects ingested enzyme 30 minutes before milk, none of the samples contained any active lactase. This demonstrated that when a lactase supplement is taken an appreciable time before food consumption, it will be destroyed by stomach acid or else it passes into the intestine prior to milk consumption. This provides no benefit to the user. In contrast, when the subjects consumed the enzyme with milk, the researchers detected strong activity at the 0 and 15 minute points. A substantial decrease had occurred by 30 minutes, and at 60 minutes virtually no active enzyme remained. Immediately after milk ingestion the average stomach pH was about 6, and at 30 minutes was about 5, in the optimal range for lactase. By 60 minutes, the pH declined to 3, which may be sufficiently acidic to inactivate this enzyme.

These results emphasize the importance of consuming lactase supplements at the immediate beginning of food consumption. They also indicate that, at least in the circumstances of the experiment, most of breakdown of lactose in the stomach occurs quickly. These results hint that, if a meal has a long duration (or contains an ice cream dessert), a second dose of supplement would be useful to fortify efficacy. As mentioned previously, some of the active lactase may pass into the more benign intestine and work during the transit to the colon. The Nagoya experiment was not able to evaluate this aspect, and the role of the small intestine in lactase supplement efficacy remains unknown.

Understanding the sites of efficacy of supplemental lactase would appear to provide opportunities for product improvements, but apparently no one has been willing to invest in this research endeavor. A number of other factors such as the presence of bile acids and digestive enzymes may also interfere with lactase efficacy, but again we know little about this area.

ADVICE FOR THE LACTOSE INTOLERANT CONSUMER

For individuals plagued by lactose intolerance symptoms, lactose-free dairy products generally offer the best solution, as there is virtually no lactose to cause problems. If someone develops symptoms after consuming lactose-free dairy products, this probably indicates an allergic or psychosomatic response. In many situations, including social gatherings, lactose-free dairy products are not available. Other than dairy avoidance, the only short-term solution is to consume tablets of a lactase enzyme supplement. Proper consumption of the supplements is crucial for efficacy. If the tablets are consumed too early, say 15 or 30 minutes before eating or drinking, the enzyme may be destroyed by gastric acidity and little functional enzyme will remain when lactose finally enters the stomach. Consuming the tablets immediately with the beginning of a meal, or within a few minutes of beginning, is probably optimal. Although swallowing or chewing tablets at the beginning of a meal may cause embarrassment to some people, or invite unwanted questioning, this is the best approach therapeutically. The enzyme and lactose will reach the stomach at much the same time, and the enzyme will benefit from the increase in stomach pH resulting from food intake. Consuming the enzyme at some time after beginning eating is also probably suboptimal, as some lactose will inevitably enter the intestine before the enzyme can attack it. This lactose will begin an uninterrupted trip to the colon, where it can wreak havoc on the individual. In addition, as mentioned previously, a second serving of lactase tablets may be useful during a long meal, or if the meal ends with a dairy dessert.

The amount of enzyme (or number of tablets) that should be consumed is also uncertain, and something that must be customized by the user. Humans differ greatly in their physiology, and the amount of enzyme that prevents symptoms in one person may be ineffective in a second person consuming the same foods. Also, the amount of lactose consumed and probably the overall nutritional content of the meal may affect efficacy. In order to achieve the best results, the user must experiment with the amount of enzyme consumed, keeping in mind the amount of dairy foods consumed and the overall structure of the meal. Keeping a diary of foods consumed, tablets ingested, and the occurrence of symptoms may help with this quest. Many people will find that some trial and error (with recordkeeping) helps to find the optimal dosing.

Most enzymes are delicate molecules, and lactase supplements are no exception. The user should handle them carefully, avoiding exposure to heat and moisture. A summer afternoon in a closed car could render supplements worthless. Similarly, purchase and shipment require attention. The user should seek high volume stores, so that product will be fresh. Internet purchases may be problematic, as a package left for hours on a hot driveway, porch, or mailbox may result in a partial or total loss of efficacy. Finally, for large quantity purchases, tablets will maintain best efficacy by refrigeration in a tightly closed container.

OTHER TREATMENT APPROACHES

Lactose free dairy products and lactase supplements are the most scientifically plausible and most commonly used approaches for preventing symptoms. Lactose free dairy appears to be the perfect solution, at least in situations where these products are available. However, other approaches are available.

As noted previously, yogurt is generally a benign food for the lactose intolerant. It could be viewed as a natural approach that combines reduced lactose levels with lactase supplementation. A portion (about 14%) of the lactose in yogurt is broken down by the streptococci and lactobacilli used to ferment yogurt. Additionally, the lactase contained in yogurt and the bacteria themselves appear to continue to breakdown lactose after yogurt consumption. Some individuals do develop symptoms from the small of lactose remaining in yogurt. For them, lactose free yogurt is available.

Other treatment approaches have been proposed (and marketed). Generally, these lack a strong base of credible supporting science, many of these approaches based on dairy and lactose adaptation theories, which Chapter 10 discussed.

One intriguing approach that is still in an early stage of development is the use of specialized prebiotics (typically fiber-like materials) to expand the number of lactose-metabolizing bacteria in the colon, or possibly the small intestine. This again is really a form of the lactose adaptation hypothesis discussed earlier.

An early stage effort in this area has indicated qualified efficacy. However, adherence to the required treatment program would be a challenge for many users.

A trial published by Dr. Dennis Savaiano of Purdue University and colleagues, and funded by Ritter Pharmaceuticals, provides details of the treatment program and its benefits.[182] The test material used is a specialized galactooligosaccharide (or GOS), which is a general term for short chains of galactose, one of the two simple sugars that make up lactose. This is essentially a specialized dietary fiber. Colon bacteria apparently metabolize GOS in a manner similar to lactose. The treatment approach in this study was complicated and would perhaps be exhausting for the consumer. It consisted initially of consuming 1.5 g of GOS per day for five days. After this, the dose increased every five days, and by the end of the 36-day treatment period users were consuming 7.5 g of GOS twice a day (or 15 g per day of supplemented dietary fiber). Subjects did not consume dairy during this 36-day period, but they could begin unrestricted use of dairy after this. Dr. Savaiano's clinical study compared lactose intolerance symptoms and breath hydrogen levels in a group that followed this regimen with GOS, and in a parallel group that received placebo. At the end of the 36-day treatment period, they evaluated with a lactose tolerance test (25 g of lactose). They repeated this test after 30 days of dairy consumption, or 66 days after GOS dosing began. There were improvements in some symptom scores for GOS, compared to the placebo. However, the decrease in breath hydrogen was minor for GOS compared to placebo, raising questions about the amount of alteration of the overall fermentation process. A substudy analyzed the bacterial DNA in fecal samples collected before GOS dosing, after the 36 days of treatment, and after the additional 30 days of dairy consumption. The levels of several species of Bifidobacterium (including B. longum, B. adolescens, and B. dentium) were significantly increased at 36 and 66 days, indicating a positive effect on this group of beneficial microorganisms.[183]

This work with a special GOS is intriguing in that it suggests that prebiotic treatment can alter the colon flora to reduce lactose intolerance symptoms. However, the researchers did not evaluate efficacy at more than 30 days after the end of treatment, and additional research is needed to determine if any colon changes are truly permanent.

SUMMARY

Scientific advances in the last century led to recognition of lactose intolerance as a specific physiological problem. Prior to this, difficulties in digesting milk were likely ascribed to vague, non-specific physiological issues. Understanding of this problem set the stage for effective treatments.

The best treatment options for sufferers of lactose intolerance are lactose-free dairy products and lactase supplements. Targeted approaches under development for altering the colon flora may offer relief, but to be effective these approaches will likely require daily ingestion of potentially large amounts of material. These are not treatments that can be turned on immediately before eating ice cream, but rather require long-term planning. Considering that compliance for taking prescription drugs for even life-threatening conditions is generally poor, it is not clear how many individuals would be motivated to adhere to an involved daily regimen.

One other aspect of lactose intolerance that could have a huge impact on treatment success for some individuals is the stress response. In some individuals, consumption of dairy is accompanied by stress over whether symptoms will follow, particularly if the occasion is outside the safety of the home. Over time, this conditioned stress response itself can cause symptoms similar to those of lactose intolerance, and successful treatment may require dealing with this stress reaction as well dealing with lactose itself. In the following chapter we will explore this intertwining of the brain and intestine in more detail.

12 LACTOSE INTOLERANCE, STRESS, AND A WHIRLPOOL OF NEGATIVE EMOTION

THE STORY TO THIS POINT IS PERHAPS TOO SIMPLE

The preceding chapters presented lactase non-persistence and lactose intolerance in terms of genetics and physiology, beginning with the DNA SNP's that render some people lactose tolerant, and then moving to the physiology of diagnosis and treatment. We have now plowed through most of our knowledge of this realm of lactase persistence and non-persistence. However, throughout these chapters the skeptical reader may have detected lurking uncertainties about the accuracy of the diagnosis and the effectiveness of treatments. For example, some people claim to be severely lactose intolerant even though they do not have increased breath hydrogen levels after lactose intake, or they show the increase in blood glucose after lactose ingestion that indicates its breakdown in the small intestine. Others claim to suffer severe symptoms after minor dairy consumption, particularly if this is in the context of stress or a disrupted lifestyle. Yet others experience symptoms of lactose intolerance after consuming tiny amounts of lactose potentially hidden in the modern diet, such as is contained as filler in a drug tablet or a minor ingredient in a salad dressing. These seemingly inexplicable situations appear to be common, and have long complicated the discussions about the prevalence and severity of lactose intolerance. Although other causes such as milk allergies may be rarely involved in these situations, it seems possible that the interactions between the brain and body often play a contributive or even causative role.

STRESS EXACERBATES GI PROBLEMS

Emotional stress may play a role in the post-dairy symptoms suffered by some individuals. Perhaps in others it may be the primary cause. Stress is involved in other GI conditions that display symptoms not too different from those of lactose intolerance. The prime example is Irritable Bowel Syndrome (IBS). This a condition is experienced by 10-20% of the population worldwide, and it affects predominantly women.[184] The occurrence of specific symptoms in the absence of any direct physical cause is often the basis for an IBS diagnosis. Essentially, this is a diagnosis by exclusion; if symptoms occur in the absence of a physical abnormality, the condition is labelled as IBS. It is often sporadic, cycling through active periods and then periods of remission. Symptoms differ greatly among patients, but frequently include diarrhea, constipation (both sometime alternating in the same person), bloating, and abdominal discomfort. Some understanding of IBS and its treatment is relevant to lactose intolerance, since both these conditions share many of the same symptoms.

INTERACTIONS OF THE BRAIN AND GI TRACT

A short detour into examining how the brain and the GI tract interact is necessary in order to understand the effects of stress on IBS, and perhaps lactose intolerance. The human brain and gut interact with each other through diverse pathways (the so called "gut-brain axis"). These brain-GI interactions involve two distinct pathways.

Afferent and efferent nerves mediate the first pathway. Afferent nerves transmit messages, often unconscious, from the various parts of the GI tract to the brain. The tissues lining the intestine are rich in nerve endings, and many types of receptors sense various aspects of the local environment and transmit information to the brain. These messages constantly update the brain on conditions such the presence of food in the stomach and the amount of distension or stretching of the intestine. These nerve endings may also transmit information about harmful or toxic material or the presence of infection. The GI tract is a large and uniquely vulnerable part of the body, and the brain requires extensive information to monitor its condition.

In response to the afferent signals, the brain fires messages back to the GI tract by a different set of nerves, the efferent nerves. These neural communications are responsible for the very short-term (seconds or minutes) control of the GI tract, and involve such things as the intensity of intestinal contractions and the rate of release of digesta from the stomach, and its passage through the intestine.

Hormones mediate the second pathway of gut-brain interactions. The brain itself produces some of these hormones, and they directly affect target sites in the body. Other hormones released from the brain trigger other organs to release additional hormones that may affect GI function. Additionally, the adrenal glands adjacent to the kidneys produce hormones that may affect the brain as well as other portions of the body. A complex interaction between the pituitary and hypothalamus of the brain, and the adrenal glands mediates the most important hormonal pathway in the GI response. This interaction leads to release of the stress hormone cortisol into the bloodstream.

CORTISOL

Cortisol is a powerful hormone that implements the body's response to the brain's perception of stress. It is the major driver of the "fight or flight" response, and it has many effects inside and outside of the GI tract. In response to the brain's perception of stress, the hypothalamus secretes corticotrophin releasing factor (CRF) into the blood. CRF triggers the pituitary to release corticotrophin to the circulation, which then stimulates the adrenal glands to release cortisol. Cortisol has wide-ranging and pronounced physiological effects that prepare the body to respond to a perceived threat. These include increased heart rate, elevated blood pressure, and increased blood glucose. In the intestine, cortisol may produce increased gut motility, which can lead to diarrhea. Also, blood supply may be redirected from the intestine and stomach to the muscles, slowing overall digestion. This shift ensures that blood is directed to muscles involved in fight or flight instead of digesting lunch. It also affects visceral sensitivity, increasing the sense of pain associated with bloating or other physical stimuli. Emerging research suggests that cortisol may even affect the composition of the gut microbiota, which could possibly affect digestion and lead to other GI symptoms. A later section of this chapter covers in more detail the overall interactions among the gut microbiome, the gut, and the brain.

STRESS AND IBS

Stress contributes to IBS severity by altering sensory perceptions from the GI tract. Input from the GI tract to the brain via afferent nerves is generally not consciously perceived. However, in IBS individuals may sense these nerve communications in the form of intermittent or constant pain. A number of factors may trigger the upregulation from an unconscious level to perceived pain, including the broad effects that stress may have on the brain. Increased perceptions of pain may occur in other parts of the body as well. In fact, stress may lead to a "generalized central pain amplification state" (a term coined by Mayer and Tillisch and skillfully described in their report).[185]

Stress and intestinal infections may interact in causing IBS symptoms. About 10% of infectious gastroenteritis patients develop IBS-like symptoms after the infection resolves. Mayer and Tillisch noted that this phenomenon is especially likely to occur in females, persons with psychosocial stress at the time of infection, and those with pre-existing anxiety and depression. This suggests that the overall emotional state may be involved in a conversion of unconscious nerve impulses into perceived pain. These post-infection symptoms are particularly likely to occur in people with a history of somatization (the conversion of anxiety into physical symptoms). These individuals may have nervous systems that are especially prone to converting normally benign nerve impulses into perceptions of pain. Bear in mind that this post-infection phenomenon may be more complicated, with other factors such as immune system upregulation possibly involved. Gastroenteritis may damage the intestinal villi where lactase is located, causing secondary lactose intolerance. Consequently, symptoms after dairy consumption could exacerbate those of IBS. Additionally, undiagnosed persistent small intestine bacterial overgrowth (SIBO) often occurs after infectious gastroenteritis, causing symptoms that may mimic both IBS and lactose intolerance.

RELEVANCE OF IBS TO LACTOSE INTOLERANCE

The most common symptoms of lactose intolerance (abundant flatulence, bloating, cramping, and diarrhea) are quite similar to those of stress and diarrheal IBS, raising the issue of whether it is possible to clearly distinguish among these conditions in a specific individual. Extensive work indicates that most IBS sufferers are not lactose intolerant. However, the reverse is certainly not true, and based on the worldwide incidence noted above one would expect that 10-20% of all lactose intolerant individuals would also suffer from IBS. The physiological effects of stress are widespread, and it seems likely that a large number of lactose intolerant individuals suffer similar effects of stress on their GI tracts.

This discussion leads to an interesting convergence of the current knowledge of these conditions. Lactose intolerant individuals suffer symptoms that derive from their inability to digest and absorb lactose. These individuals also often have a long history of battling the symptoms of this condition, which unfortunately may develop in public places or other unaccommodating surroundings. When these individuals later confront dairy products in similar circumstances, recollections of this unpleasant history may be sufficient to stimulate a stress response. The individual recalls memories of unpleasant experiences, triggering a stress response in the brain that affects the entire body, including the intestine. Since stress may cause increased visceral sensitivity and motility as well as diarrhea, these symptoms may overlay or amplify any symptoms caused directly by the physiological effects of lactose.

In individuals who lack lactase, the response to lactose ingestion varies greatly, ranging from no symptoms to full force outbreaks of pain, gas, and diarrhea. Even for a given individual, the response to dairy consumption may vary widely from day to day. Overall dietary intake, the condition of the GI tract, and emotional state likely influence this response. The perceptions of the individual derive from the physiological effects of lactose, the manner in which the brain processes afferent nerve inputs from the intestine, and emotional concerns. Such concerns include the broad issues imposed by the individual's entire life, as well as more immediate factors related to the potentially painful and embarrassing effects of lactose intolerance.

It is easy to envision that in some individuals a downward spiral occurs, in which physiological effects of lactose intolerance become magnified by a conditioned stress response based on bad memories from prior bouts of lactose intolerance. The stress response may become so pronounced that it surpasses the direct effects of lactose intolerance. In these individuals, the stress response may cause the ingestion of seemingly innocuous amounts of lactose, such as in coffee creamer or hard cheeses, to be followed by GI symptoms. This may also account for reports of people developing intolerance symptoms after consuming lactose-free milk. Similarly, in individuals who suffer short bouts of secondary lactose intolerance, they may retain these stress-related GI symptoms even after they return to normal lactase production.

The interaction of stress and lactose intolerance are difficult to study, and no published research has sought to separate the direct symptoms of lactose intolerance from the symptoms related to dairy ingestion stress or IBS. The role of stress in lactose intolerance is perhaps the least understood aspect of this condition. Hopefully this area will receive attention in the future.

IMPLICATIONS FOR COPING WITH LACTOSE INTOLERANCE

The preceding discussion hypothesizes that the symptoms of lactose intolerance, at least in some individuals, is more than just a painful response to the bacterial fermentation products of lactose. This broader view incorporates the psychological response to consumption of dairy, or even the thought of consuming dairy foods. Prior bad experiences can prime an individual to experience fear and apprehension when ingesting the same dairy foods that have previously caused problems. This may be part of a more primitive aversion system that helps animals to avoid consuming foods that have been previously associated with illness. Such aversion could unleash a flood of stress hormones like cortisol that can directly cause some GI symptoms. The affected individual may experience the ensuing symptoms with increased intensity, since the individual is already primed to expect GI discomfort.

Although there is essentially no research on the role of stress reduction in managing lactose intolerance, there is extensive work on behavioral approaches to dealing with the similar symptoms of IBS. Thus, it is intriguing to identify what has been effective in IBS, and to pose these approaches as having potential benefits in lactose intolerance. Some behavioral techniques demonstrate effectiveness in mitigating IBS, and perhaps could also provide useful tools for those with lactose intolerance.

Negative thoughts, harmful emotions, and excessive stress may exacerbate IBS symptoms. Researchers at the University of North Carolina at Chapel Hill have demonstrated that limited psychological interventions can lead to major improvements in perceived IBS symptoms.[186] A trial conducted by Dr. Susan Gaylord and colleagues used mindfulness meditation techniques that emphasize mind-body interactions, such as viewing the body's activity in an objective, non-judgmental manner. These techniques were based on a highly regarded approach developed by Dr. Jon Kabat-Zinn at the University of Massachusetts, and they place emphasis on living in the present moment, instead of rehashing the past or visioning the future. The Chapel Hill team recruited local female IBS subjects who were currently under physician care for their condition. For the randomly selected mindfulness group, they conducted intensive group training in these techniques for two months. They placed the randomly selected control subjects in an IBS support group that received a similar intensity of training for two months. The control support group did not receive training in the mindfulness techniques. Earlier work had shown that the training received by the control group provided benefits to IBS patients. Members of the two groups performed self-assessment scales for IBS symptom severity just after completion of training, and again at three months after training. Just after the training, the mindfulness group reported a 26% reduction in symptoms, compared to just 6% for the control support group. The improvement was even greater at three months after the end of treatment, with the mindfulness group showing a 38% reduction, in contrast to 12% for the support group members. The mindfulness group had significant improvements in abdominal pain frequency, and the degree to which bowel symptoms interfered with normal life. This study indicates that a non-pharmacological behavioral intervention can be substantially effective in reducing IBS symptoms. One must wonder if a similar program targeting the stress associated with lactose intolerance could also reduce the severity of symptoms. Hopefully someday such a study will be conducted.

IBS has a tremendous detrimental effect on the quality of life (QOL). In many individuals, it appears that the fear of GI symptoms, rather than the symptoms themselves, is the strongest factor in the negative effect of IBS on QOL.[187] For these individuals, the earliest signs of GI symptoms raise concerns of an imminent threat of overwhelming distress. This induces fear-provoking anxiety that can further exacerbate their severity, likely at least partially due to cortisol release. To some extent, the fear response to IBS symptoms reflects a general disposition of these individuals to experience fear in stressful situations. Therefore the fear of symptoms magnifies the effects that IBS has on the individual's life, and the difficulty in working through these fears sets up a downward spiral of negative expectations. The role of fear in the impact that IBS has on individual has applicability to lactose intolerance, and diminishing the sense of fear experienced by lactose intolerance sufferers might improve their overall ability to adapt to this condition.

Lactose intolerance, on first appearances at the beginning of this book, seemed to be a simple physiological response to lactose intake in people who do not produce intestinal lactase. In reality, the condition appears more complex with strong interactions with an individual's overall personality and behavior. The stresses associated with the symptoms of lactose intolerance can provide negative feedback to the brain and body, exacerbating both the severity of the symptoms and the overall level of distress. For some individuals, use of effective dietary supplements such as lactase tablets may not fully control symptoms. For them, use of the behavioral techniques such as mindfulness meditation that provide significant relief in IBS may serve a role in more fully controlling their symptoms. The specific tools developed for controlling IBS, as well as more generic methods for promoting relaxation and reducing the negative effects of stress, are readily available. Committed individuals may do well to explore their effectiveness in lactose intolerance. A brief book by Dr. Jeffrey Lackner describes a highly researched mindfulness-based approach for treating IBS, and the techniques it contains may be of use to those with lactose intolerance.[188]

INTERACTIONS AMONG THE MICROBIOME, GI TRACT, AND BRAIN: IMPLICATIONS FOR LACTOSE INTOLERANCE?

An effect of cortisol on the composition of the gut microbiota was alluded to earlier in this chapter. The actual situation is far more complex, and research over the last few years indicates intricate interactions between the brain and the intestinal microbiome pseudo-organ. The brain-gut axis may be more accurately described as the brain-gut-biome axis. Since these interactions appear to involve stress and other aspects of the emotional state, they could affect perceptions of lactose intolerance. Additionally, in lactose intolerant individuals, consuming lactose results in a large input of a prebiotic-like material into the lower GI tract. This could alter the gut microbiota, possibly unleashing effects on both mind and body.

The effects of stress on the makeup of the human gut microbiome have received relatively little attention, but some animal studies indicate that stress can induce significant alterations. Bharwani and colleagues used a model involving stressed mice to evaluate effects on the microbiome.[189] They compared the gut microbiome of chronic "socially defeated" mice and control animals. They created socially defeated mice by subjecting them to multiple sessions of cohabiting a small cage with a highly dominant aggressor mouse of the same sex, which is apparently an extremely stressful social interaction for mice. The stressed mice had a decrease in overall diversity of the colon bacteria, compared to controls. In addition, the defeated mice had a decreased overall richness of the microbial community with lower occurrences of rare species. The stressed mice had altered levels of some modulators of the immune system, such as interleukin-6, which the authors hypothesized as underlying the microbiome shift. Thus, stress not only affects virtually every part of the body, but also may even extend to the microorganisms living in the intestine. A large amount of recent work demonstrates that changes in the microbiome can influence overall health, and these stress-induced microbiota changes could have unknown consequences.[190]

INTERPLAY BETWEEN EMOTION AND THE GUT MICROBIOME

In contrast to the limited information on the effects of the brain on gut bacteria, a recent outpouring of research has focused on the potential of probiotic bacteria to positively affect behavior and cognition; these organisms have been dubbed "psychobiotics."

Intriguing findings from investigations in mice suggest that the gut bacteria can play a role in modulating anxiety levels.[191] Researchers at McMaster University in Hamilton, Ontario, induced intestinal irritation in mice, which resulted in anxiety-like symptoms (it is of course not possible to ask mice directly about their emotional state, but anxiety can be inferred from their behavior). Mice treated with the oral probiotic *Bifidobacterium longum* NCC3001 lost their anxiety symptoms, and behaved like non-anxious, untreated control mice. The vagus nerve carries messages from the intestine to the brain, and proved key to the anti-anxiety effect of the probiotic. If the scientists surgically severed the vagus in mice with GI irritation, the mice were no longer cured of their anxiety by *B. longum* treatment. This suggests that the probiotic reduces anxiety by decreasing the excitability of enteric neurons, the neurons that send signals from the gut to the brain. These findings raise the possibility that in humans, alterations of the gut bacterial populations could affect stress-related symptoms like anxiety. Diet powerfully influences the intestinal microbial balance. It is possible that, in people with underlying GI distress, alterations of perceptions of pain and anxiety could follow dietary changes. An interplay between the gut microbiome and anxiety could be responsible for reports by many individuals that their IBS symptoms are strongly responsive to changes in diet.

Probiotic researchers at University College in Cork, Ireland, compared the bacterial composition of fecal samples obtained from a group of depressed patients (recruited from outpatient psychiatric clinics) and a matched set of controls.[192] Compared to the normal controls, depressed people had a decrease in overall richness of the microbiome, as defined by a decrease in the total number of species present. In addition, they found that depressed people had a significant reduction in number of bacteria in the *Prevotella* group. They also had increased levels of inflammatory factors in the blood, and elevated morning cortisol levels. Interestingly, dietary fiber intake in the depressed was lower than in normal individuals, and within the depressed group there was a strong correlation between decreasing fiber intake levels and increased severity of depression, as measured by the Beck Depression Scale. Of course, this is merely correlation, and it is possible that increasing depression results in decreased consumption of high fiber foods.

Depression in humans thus appears in at least some cases to be causally associated with alterations in the gut microbiota. Intriguingly, transfer of the microbiome from depressed humans to rats induces behavior resembling depression in the rats. In a clever experiment, these same Irish researchers developed a procedure for introducing the microflora of depressed humans into rats. Initially they used an intense regimen of antibiotic treatment to greatly reduce the gut bacteria population in a group of rats. They divided these microbe-depleted rats into two populations. One received an oral gavage of bacteria extracted from feces of three depressed men, and the second group received a similar gavage obtained from three otherwise similar normal men. The scientists performed these oral inoculations daily for three days, then twice weekly. The rats inoculated with microbiota from depressed men developed anxiety-like behavior, such as decreased activity in a maze test, and avoiding time in open areas. Rats inoculated with samples from the control human subjects did not demonstrate such altered behavior. Notably the two groups did not differ in levels of corticosterone, which is the rat hormone analogous to human cortisol. After these fecal inoculations the two rat groups also differed in profiles of fecal microbiota, although the differences did not closely match those observed between the microbiomes of depressed and normal humans. These results suggest that the microbiota are linked with depression and, at least in rats, the implanting of the microbiome of depressed humans can induce depressive symptoms. This intriguing work suggests that the microbiome may partly cause human anxiety and stress. It is easy to imagine that, in the appropriate people, this could affect the severity of lactose intolerance symptoms.

This Irish work showed that transfer of fecal bacteria from depressed humans to rats resulted in the rats displaying depression-like symptoms. Other evidence indicates that a probiotic milk, a much more appealing food, can affect the human brain.[193] A group of women received a fermented milk containing a blend of prebiotics (including bifidobacteria, lactobacilli, and streptococci). One control group received an identical tasting milk without probiotics, and a second control group received no treatment at all. Functional magnetic resonance imaging (fMRI) was performed on the subjects' brains before treatment, and again at the end of the four-week treatment period. The fMRI measured the subjects' brain activity in response to viewing pictures of emotional faces, and it also evaluated resting brain activity. Consumption of the fermented milk (but not the other two treatments) resulted in changes in mid-brain activity associated with decreased anxiety responses. Each subject's emotional state was also measured with questionnaires during the study. The women receiving fermented milk did not report any changes in anxiety and depression, but the women were in generally good emotional health at the beginning of the study. This study indicates that probiotic intake can affect brain activity, but this work needs to be repeated in subjects suffering from anxiety, stress, and depression to determine if the probiotics can improve mental health.

Prebiotics are dietary fibers that cause proliferation of beneficial colon bacteria, as discussed in Chapter 10. These also appear to be capable of affecting the brain and behavior. Researchers at Oxford University in England recruited human volunteers to drink a beverage containing either one of two prebiotics (galactooligosaccharide (known as GOS), and fructooligosaccharide (FOS)), or a starch placebo.[194] In this double-blind test, separate groups of volunteers consumed one of these treatments for three weeks. Salivary cortisol concentrations during the first hour after morning rising were measured, along with a number of behavioral responses related to depression. Cortisol levels declined significantly in the group that received GOS, but not in the groups receiving the FOS prebiotic or the starch placebo.

To evaluate depression, the researchers monitored subjects' reaction times to positive and negative words. One of 60 positive or 60 negative words appeared briefly (about 1/60 of second) on a computer screen, interspersed with a mask of various other words and keyboard symbols. Subjects had to record the appearance of a positive or negative word by pressing one of two keys. Reaction times in responding to these words provided a measure of depression. In subjects who had received GOS, there was a significant decrease in reaction time to positive words, in comparison to subjects receiving placebo. The administration of antidepressant drugs such as citalopram (a serotonin reuptake inhibitor) and the benzodiazepine diazepam have similar effects. Thus, at least by this measure, the GOS treatment appeared to have a measurable antidepressant effect in addition to the observed decrease in the stress hormone cortisol.

These investigators also examined the effects of these two prebiotics in rats. GOS ingestion resulted in a pronounced increase in the colon bifidobacteria population. In contrast, FOS has a smaller effect on bifidobacteria, and starch had no effect. Thus the human effects of GOS in decreasing a stress hormone (cortisol) and improving sense of well-being could result from its boosting the bifidobacteria population.

The importance of the gut microbiome to human health has received increasing attention over the last few years. The concept of psychobiotics is even more recent, and the emerging data indicate that the microbiome could have multiple effects, both good and bad, on mental health. The idea that colon bacteria could affect the functioning of the human brain to alter perceptions of anxiety would have seemed very far-fetched a few years ago. However, an outpouring of research from credible scientists at prestigious institutions is starting to unravel this unusual function of colon bacteria. Possibly increasing learnings in this area will change our understandings of how the brain functions, and its impact on conditions impacted by stress, such as lactose intolerance. Perhaps in the future, altering the composition of the colon bacteria may play a role in optimizing mental health.

SUMMARY

The classic view of lactose intolerance is that it is a simple biological process. According to this view, in the absence of intestinal lactase, lactose passes through the small intestine unaltered and enters the colon, where it causes osmotic diarrhea, and its fermentation by bacteria results in flatulence and cramping. A more encompassing hypothesis is that intolerance symptoms derive from both this physiological basis and a stress response by the sufferer. This stress may increase over time, and in susceptible people each round of lactose intolerance symptoms (exacerbated by this stress response) may further amplify the severity of this psychobiological problem.

Assuming that this hypothesis has some value, stress reduction techniques or steps to undo this negative conditioning could play a role in ameliorating intolerance symptoms, of course in combination with restrained intake of high lactose foods or the use of lactase supplements. Research on applications of stress reduction techniques to control IBS provide a useful analogy.

The colon microbiome is under intense investigation for its effects on overall human physiology, and emerging science indicates that these colon bacteria can affect the behaviors of both animals and humans. It is not farfetched to think that in the future probiotics or prebiotics may play a role in mitigating both the physiological and psychological aspects of lactose intolerance.

13 DO THE LACTOSE INTOLERANT REALLY NEED DAIRY? IMPLICATIONS OF DAIRY AVOIDANCE

The previous chapters dealt with the causes of lactose tolerance and intolerance. The genetic changes that result in adult lactase persistence have certainly provided a selective advantage in populations that raise dairy animals (although the identity of this advantage remains uncertain). Dairy products play a substantial nutritional role in these populations. However, the overall health role of dairy products is less clear. A number of scientists and health experts have maintained that dairy, particularly milk, is so important to good health and nutrition that just about everyone should consume it. In the United States the dairy industry and the USDA have long supported this view, and USDA guidelines call for three daily servings of dairy. The nutritional benefits of dairy are indisputable. However, humans survived for many millennia before dairy animals were domesticated, and today much of the world's population does not consume milk after childhood. These people apparently achieve nutritional adequacy from their dairy-free diets. Some low dairy consuming populations lead the world for longevity and fitness late in life. A prime example is Okinawa, where the traditional diet contains little or dairy. This diet is largely plant-based, with the sweet potato as a major source of energy intake.[195] Okinawans have the world's longest life expectancy. Clearly humans thrived before dairy animals were domesticated and dairy consumption is not essential for good health and longevity.

This chapter will explore two components of dairy widely recognized for their nutritional benefits: protein and calcium. We will address protein first, since this is the simpler story. Following this, we will examine the more complicated and controversial role of dairy calcium in maintaining bone health.

THE ROLE OF DAIRY PROTEIN IN MAINTAINING MUSCLE AND MOBILITY

Milk and dairy are renowned as excellent protein sources, and for some they are a key food for obtaining adequate protein intake. In the United States, the recommended adult daily intake of protein is 0.8 g per kg of body weight. Most individuals on a Western diet readily achieve this intake. However, increasing evidence indicates that this level of protein intake may not be sufficient for maintaining health in older adults. Older adults may actually need about 1.0 to 1.2 g per kg body weight, or up to 50% more than this recommendation.[196] A weight of 70 kg is commonly used to represent the average adult weight, including men and women (given the epidemic of overweight and obesity, this value understates the weight of much of the population). However, based on the 70 kg value, "recommended" daily protein intake for the general population would be 56 g and 70-84 g for older people. For reasons described below, this protein intake should be evenly divided among three or four meals each day. The causes for increased protein needs in the elderly are not clear, but may include less efficient digestion and a need for higher blood levels of some amino acids to trigger synthesis of skeletal muscle. Muscle mass inexorably decreases with age, and low protein intake exacerbates this process.

Sarcopenia is the medical term for this age-related loss of skeletal muscle. It has an onset in middle age, and accelerates with increasing age. After 50, people generally lose 0.5-1.0% of muscle per year. In addition to this insidious gradual loss, disease or periods of immobility result in rapid losses from unused muscles. Even with a later high protein diet and appropriate exercise, older people may not be able to restore this lost muscle mass. Unlike fats and carbohydrates, the body has no reservoir of protein. When protein intake is less than the body's need, the depletion of skeletal muscle fills this deficit, leading to sarcopenia.

Sarcopenia can lead to a deterioration in overall health. "Frailty" is a term for physical weakness or deterioration, and of course has more precise scientific definitions. Clinicians consider a patient frail if three of the following five criteria are present: exhaustion, weakness, low physical activity, slow walking speed, and weight loss (each of these criteria has its own detailed definition).[197] Several studies to be reviewed shortly do in fact indicate that increased dairy protein intake is associated with greater muscle mass and decreased frailty in older people. Thus, dairy can mitigate sarcopenia and its deleterious consequences.

Skeletal muscle mass is in a constant state of fluctuation. During periods of fasting, muscle is broken down to provide amino acids for the body's needs. Consumption of suitable and adequate protein restores this lost muscle. With aging, the rate of muscle synthesis decreases after protein consumption, and over time this leads to the decreased muscle mass associated with frailty. Specific amino acids activate muscle protein synthesis, and the levels needed to trigger muscle formation increases with age. This muscle anabolic resistance can be somewhat overcome by higher levels of protein intake, particularly protein sources that are high in these essential amino acids. This amino acid effect can be saturated, and beyond a certain level further protein intake does little or nothing to boost muscle synthesis. For this reason, the optimal strategy for reducing sarcopenia is to maintain an adequate protein intake, and to divide this intake fairly equally among multiple meals. This flies in the face of the common practice of consuming much a day's protein at a single meal (usually dinner).

Dairy in general is a good source of the essential amino acids needed to trigger muscle synthesis. In support of this, whey protein is the test material used in many of the human trials investigating the effects of dietary protein on muscle synthesis. Whey protein has high levels of leucine, the primary amino acid that triggers muscle synthesis after protein consumption.[198] Although whey protein powder has some unique advantages because of its low fat level and rapid digestibility, most other dairy foods with high protein content are also rich in essential amino acids, including leucine.

Elevated intake of low fat dairy foods appears to delay the onset of some measures of frailty in the elderly. Spanish researchers measured the amount of dairy consumed by 1871 individuals 60 and older (average of 69), and compared this intake to appearance of indicators of frailty two to four years later.[199] During a mean follow up period of 3½ years, 7% of all subjects became frail. Study results indicated that, in comparison to people who consumed less than one serving per week of low fat milk or yogurt, those who consumed seven or more servings of low fat dairy per week had a statistically significant decrease in onset of slow walking speed or weight loss. This overall decrease in frailty onset in the high dairy consumers was a remarkable almost 50%. In contrast, a similar analysis of whole fat milk consumption did not show any difference in the onset of frailty between high and low dairy consumption groups. The reason for the differences in the low and high fat dairy groups is unclear. Perhaps in the whole fat dairy group, saturated fat intake or additional calories somehow negated the beneficial effect of dairy in preventing frailty. Alternatively, perhaps these results reflect differences between these two populations. Health professionals and government agencies generally recommend low fat dairy products. The low fat dairy group may have been more health conscious overall. In addition to consuming low fat dairy, they may have pursued other recommended behaviors that limited development of frailty. Although these researchers attempted to incorporate obvious confounding lifestyle factors into their statistical analysis, correlation and causation are always difficult to distinguish in prospective cohort studies like this.

An analysis of dairy intake by individuals over 40 enrolled in the Framingham Offspring Study (a second generation follow-up of the original Framingham cohort) also showed a protective effect of dairy.[200] In this study, men and women who daily consumed more than 2 or 1.75 servings of dairy respectively had about a 22% decrease in risk of developing physical disabilities related frailty, compared to those who consumed less than one serving per day. These disabilities included difficulties with distance walking, vigorous housework, and carrying heavy objects. Unfortunately, this analysis did not separate low and high fat dairy consumption, so it could not confirm the specific protective effect of low fat dairy observed in the Spanish research.

A recent meta-analysis of clinical trials evaluating the effects of protein in preserving physical function confirms the beneficial role of elevated protein intakes, including dairy. Coelho-Júnior and colleagues evaluated seven studies involving 8754 older adults (>60) from six countries.[201] Note that this analysis considered data on total protein intake, not specifically dairy. Subjects were sorted into a very high protein intake group (1.2 g or more of protein/kg/day), high protein (1.0 g) or low protein (less than 0.8 g). Individuals in the two high protein groups showed superior leg function in comparison to the low protein group, as measured by walking speed and knee extension strength. Although this analysis had the benefit of pooling data from several studies meeting strict design criteria, some individual studies did not support this conclusion. This may once again reflect inadequate study design, or the general vagaries of nutrition research.

These results on the role of dairy in reducing frailty and sarcopenia are intriguing, but determining the optimal intake of dairy protein for older people requires much more work. In particular, the Spanish study that showed a major benefit of low fat dairy on reducing frailty, as compared to no effect with high fat dairy consumption, needs to be replicated and expanded.

Given the potential benefit of dairy protein and the human and economic impact of frailty, this topic deserves more attention. This is in contrast to the role of dairy in bone health. For this topic, a huge volume of sometimes contradictory research is already available. The next section will wade into this difficult area.

SUMMARY AND GUIDANCE ON MUSCLE HEALTH

In most developed societies, people are living longer, and the health consequences of aging are becoming more of a problem for both the individual and society. Health professionals recognize that maintaining adequate muscle mass results in improved mobility, reduced propensity for falls, avoidance of institutionalization, and increased longevity.[202] Although increased protein intake appears to be generally beneficial, high protein intake may contribute to renal function decline in individuals with pre-existing renal disease.[203] This population should be cautious about high levels of protein.

Returning to the question posed at the beginning of this chapter, the available evidence supports a strong role for low-fat dairy products (particularly whey protein) in maintaining muscle mass and avoiding frailty. Older people in general need more protein, and dairy is a convenient way to fortify the diet. Although dairy avoiders can likely obtain optimal protein intake from other sources, this approach requires careful diet planning and has disadvantages. Plant proteins tend to be low in the amino acids most effective in stimulating muscle synthesis, especially in comparison to whey protein, and their slower digestibility may result in blood levels too low to trigger optimal muscle synthesis. Thus, older individuals (over 50) can likely derive a substantial health benefit from low fat dairy. This is significant because currently there are no approved drugs for preventing or reducing sarcopenia. The only preventative strategy is a healthy diet, preferably in combination with rigorous exercise or weight bearing exercise.

THE ROLE OF CALCIUM IN BONE HEALTH OVER THE LIFESPAN

Bone health is one of the most commonly stated reasons for the necessity of dairy intake, and it is important to analyze the relationship between increased dairy intake and improved bone health. Before beginning this analysis, it must be reiterated that the lactose intolerant can obtain these nutritional benefits by consuming dairy products such as hard cheese, lactase-treated milk and dairy, and unpasteurized yogurt. These products will not cause GI distress in most intolerant consumers. There is no need to consume lactose-containing fluid milk to obtain the nutritional benefits of dairy.

Calcium is an element essential for a strong skeleton. Dairy products are an excellent source, and in many Western diets they are the principal source of calcium. The dairy industry has persistently exploited this relationship, and the importance of dairy in achieving adequate calcium intake and strong bones is ingrained in both the lay population and the nutrition community. Bones contain 99% of all the calcium in the body. Calcium intake from dairy during childhood does play an important role in building strong bones and teeth. Adults are also admonished to consume milk and dairy as a way of maintaining bones and preventing fractures, particularly in the later years. However, it bears repeating that in many parts of the world post-weaning children consume little or no dairy, yet mature into adults with quite adequate bone structure.

The importance of calcium intake during childhood has often been cited as a reason why lactose intolerant individuals should consume dairy,[204,205] but what is beneficial to children may not necessarily benefit adults. Health advocates also often place particular emphasis on calcium and dairy intake for post-menopausal women, for whom loss of bone calcium often leads to osteoporosis and bone fractures. In light of the frequent invocation of calcium as a reason for adult dairy intake by the lactose intolerant, it is worthwhile to consider the science supporting the contention that dairy intake can mitigate development of osteoporosis. This degenerative condition is manifested first by decreased bone mineral density (BMD) and then by occurrence of fractures. BMD is largely a measure of the calcium content of bones, and many dairy advocates emphasize its effects on BMD. Part of this emphasis may lie in the fact that BMD is relatively easy to measure. In science, easily measured parameters often receive an exaggerated importance. Unfortunately, an effect on BMD does not necessarily extend to the benefit that really matters, decreased late-life fractures, especially hip fractures. Among the elderly, fractures of the hip and spine tend to draw most attention. These are debilitating, and difficult to heal, and their occurrence often foreshadows impending mortality.

BONE CALCIUM OVER THE HUMAN LIFESPAN

Before delving into the science of calcium and bone health, it is worthwhile to explore the changes in bones over a human lifespan. During childhood, bone mass is low and bones are relatively fragile, as evidenced by the high frequency of fractures in children. The time of peak bone building is the years just following puberty, but additional bone mass accumulates through the later teen years and into the twenties. Peak bone mass is achieved late in the third decade of life, and BMD decreases inexorably after this. With extensive loss of BMD, fracture risk increases. Weakened bones in combination with deteriorating balance account for the drastic increase in fracture risk in the elderly. Achieving peak BMD in these younger years helps protect against later osteoporosis and fracture risk. That said, lifestyle and dietary habits during the later years are perhaps of greater importance. Of course, genetics also play a largely uncontrollable role in late life bone health. For women, menopause and the loss of estrogen trigger an accelerated rate of calcium loss from bones and decreased BMD.[206]

During pregnancy and nursing, the mother's bones serve as a source of calcium for the skeleton of the growing fetus and infant. These effects of pregnancy and lactation on BMD are complex, and as noted in an earlier chapter the emergence of persistence SNP's may have allowed women to more readily consume milk. This increased calcium intake may have resulted in more frequent healthy pregnancies and infants. Perhaps this was a selective factor in the rapid expansion of these SNP's in some dairying populations.

As noted, almost all of the body's calcium is in the skeleton. Stripping this element from the mother's bones partially fills the calcium needs of a growing fetus. During pregnancy, 2-3% of the maternal calcium store transfers to the developing fetus. After birth the growing baby also needs calcium for the developing skeleton, and each day nursing moves about 300-400 mg of calcium from the mother's bones to the infant. Over the duration of lactation, about a 4-7% loss of calcium occurs in the mother's lumbar spine and the neck of the femur, sites that are often scanned to measure BMD. However, after weaning the maternal skeleton rebounds, and 12-24 months later calcium generally returns to the original level. There is considerable variation among human studies on the observed rate of this post-weaning rebound. This could reflect differences in diet, lifestyle, and perhaps vitamin D levels among the tested populations. A systematic review of this area by researchers at the University of Tehran suggested that pregnancy might have a long-term protective effect for bones, particularly if the mother nursed the newborns.[207] Unfortunately, the following recent analysis of an American population did not support this finding.

A research consortium analyzed data from a subset of postmenopausal women in the Women's Health Initiative who underwent repeated BMD testing.[208] These women were 50-79 years at the beginning of the evaluation, and the researchers monitored them for BMD and fractures for about the following nine years. These scientists reported that pregnancy history, including total number of pregnancies and length of lactation had no later effect on fracture risk, including hip fractures. This analysis based on an American population indicates that cycling of calcium in and out of bones during the childbearing years apparently does not have a long-term impact, positive or negative, on bone strength.

EFFECTS OF DAIRY ON THE RISK OF FRACTURES: CONFUSION AND LACK OF CLARITY

Despite its possible benefit to BMD, the teaching that adult dairy intake will ward off fractures later in life remains a debatable hypothesis. Clinical trials to test this hypothesis directly are likely infeasible due to the large number of subjects that would be required, a trial length of many years or decades, and the impossibility of placebo blinding for dairy products. Therefore, this analysis must rely on the epidemiological literature, particularly longitudinal studies that follow the lives and health of people for decades. Some of these studies have compared the health status of otherwise similar populations that consume varying amounts of dairy. Most of these reports have found that fluid milk intake, as well as cheese and other dairy products, do not provide protection against fractures. However, some studies have found a protective benefit. Yogurt and other fermented milk products are potentially different, and may confer some advantage.[209] The following paragraphs summarize a few of the key studies involving milk and non-fermented dairy, including one that does indicate a slight protective effect of milk drinking.

Overall, the available science does support a role for dairy in maintaining BMD, but the benefits of dairy for fracture prevention (what really matters) are more equivocal. Dairy intake increases BMD in some groups, and under some conditions. An analysis of data from the Framingham Study provides insight.[210] This pioneering epidemiological study that commenced in 1948 has followed for decades the health of an original group of 5200 residents of Framingham, Massachusetts, and many of their descendants. Data from this study were used to compare consumption of various forms of dairy and BMD in an elderly population (age range 76 to 93; mean age of 75 years). Generally, amount of dairy intake was not significantly associated with BMD, nor with changes in BMD over the preceding four years. However, in a subgroup of vitamin D supplement users there was a BMD benefit of dairy at some bone locations. Humans normally absorb only a portion of the calcium in dairy, and adequate vitamin D levels increase this absorption. This perhaps explains why only vitamin D supplement users obtained a dairy BMD benefit. Much of the population of non-tropical areas is chronically vitamin D deficient, and at the latitude of Framingham a combination of bad weather and limited sunshine for much of the year reduces the production of vitamin D in sunlight-exposed skin. Optimal calcium absorption in Framingham may have only occurred in vitamin D supplements users. Although milk in many countries, including the United States, is fortified with vitamin D, in a normal diet this source alone is not sufficient to achieve adequate levels. Prevention of rickets in children served as the basis, many decades ago, for the US fortification level, which does not reflect currently recognized levels for maximal health. The Framingham results do indicate that the relationship between dairy and BMD is not straightforward, and other powerful factors may be involved.

Similarly, a 1998 analysis of data from the Nurses' Health Study raised early concerns about the bone protective effect of dairy consumption.[211] This study, initiated in 1976, enrolled married registered nurses from eleven states. Data from about 78,000 participants were analyzed for the relationship between the amount milk consumed and incidence of forearm and hip fractures. The nurses were 35 to 60 years old at first collection of fracture incidence, and researchers collected data for 12 more years. Women in the lowest quartile of milk intake consumed one glass or less per week; in contrast, those in the highest quartile consumed two or more glasses per day. Higher milk intake had no protective effect on preventing either type of fracture. A subanalysis limited to women over 60, who have a much higher fracture incidence, yielded similar results. In contrast to the lack of protective effect for adult milk consumption, recalled intake of milk during adolescence showed a positive trend between high milk consumption during these bone-forming years and decreased fracture incidence during later adult life. A subsequent analysis of 22 years of data from the same group included a much larger number of fractures because of the increasing age of the nurses.[212] Unfortunately, this more recent study did not show any protective effect of teenage milk consumption on hip fracture incidence late in life. Of course, the accuracy of dietary recollections from up to one-half century earlier could compromise the data on reported milk intake; many people would have trouble recalling what they ate for lunch last week.

In Sweden a massive study using a government database to evaluate the effect of milk intake on fractures in men and women yielded similar results.[213] This study evaluated 61,433 women who ranged in age from 39 to 74 at baseline. The subjects completed a food frequency questionnaire at baseline, and Swedish scientists evaluated this population 20 years later for survival and incidence of all fractures, with a separate measurement of hip fractures. Similarly, they evaluated these same measures after eleven years in 45,339 men (45-79 at baseline) who had completed food questionnaires. In the analysis, they divided the men and women into four categories based on daily milk intake. Subjects in the lowest intake quartile consumed less than 200g per day (about 7 ounces, or less than a cup). The highest intake quartile consumed 600 or more grams per day, or about 3 cups or more. They reported results separately by sex, and found that the rates of total fractures and hip fractures at all four levels of milk intake were basically the same. Thus for a large group of Swedish men and women, increased milk intake was not associated with any protection against fractures, including those of the hip. A more troubling observation was that, for both sexes, increased milk consumption was associated with increased overall mortality, and increased death from cardiovascular disease. These milk-associated mortality increases were greater in women than in men. Some of these researchers later conducted a meta-analysis of all studies evaluating the relationship between dairy consumption and death from all causes, as well as from heart disease and cancer.[214] This broader analysis did not show any association between the amount of dairy consumption and death from all causes, or any effect of dairy intake on heart disease and cancer. Perhaps the earlier report was merely a spurious finding. As we have seen before, such conflicting results are annoyingly common in the nutrition literature.

A separate meta-analysis of prospective trials examining the potential for milk consumption to reduce hip fractures also showed no benefit for women.[215] This analysis pooled data from seven prospective studies in multiple countries, and involved about 200,000 women followed for periods of six and one-half to 26 years. Results showed no protective effect of milk consumption on reducing hip fractures in older women, even if they consumed three or more glasses per day. A smaller study in men showed a possible small trend toward protection.

The Framingham Study has been in progress for decades, and researchers continue to analyze the massive amount of data in many ways. One investigation focused on dairy intake, BMD, and hip fractures in the original cohort individuals in their later years.[216] A group of 764 surviving members aged from 68 to 96 (mean of 76) in 1988-1989 was followed for occurrence of hip fractures for up to 20 additional years. Dietary intake data were used to divide subjects into tertiles based on milk consumption. The lowest consumed less than one glass per week, the medium group consumed between one and seven, and the highest consumed greater than seven glasses. There was a trend toward reduced hip fractures in the two higher groups of milk consumption, compared to the group that consumed less than one glass per week. However, this trend did not reach statistical significance. The incidence of hip fractures in this population was high because of advancing age, with about one in eight participants suffering a hip fracture during the study. Many of the subjects had taken a vitamin D supplement. A separate analysis of these supplement users similarly did not show a significant benefit of milk consumption in reducing hip fractures.

Finally, another massive analysis by Dr. Diane Feskanich and colleagues in the Nutrition Department at Harvard University evaluated the effects of milk consumption on hip fractures.[217] This study used data from about 80,000 women in the Nurses' Health Study and 43,000 men in the Health Professionals Follow-up Study. This analysis found a modest effect of milk drinking on decreasing hip fracture. Each serving of milk per day was associated with statistically significant 8% reduction in hip fracture. These results are somewhat at odds with the other studies, and provide strong support for a fracture-protection benefit for late-life milk consumption.

A fact relevant to this controversy is that in the US milk by law is fortified with vitamin D. In contrast Sweden, the site of one of the large negative studies, does not have mandatory vitamin D fortification. Thus the protective benefit in the Harvard analysis may have resulted from both the calcium and vitamin D content of milk. However, as noted earlier, the amount of vitamin D obtained from dairy alone is not sufficient to achieve what are currently considered optimal levels. Likely more large studies on fractures will be reported in the future, and hopefully they will incorporate vitamin D intakes and blood level analyses.

In summary, numerous reports have examined effects of dairy on fracture incidence, generally with negative or equivocal results. Although the nutritional profiles of milk and other dairy products suggest that there should be a fracture reduction benefit, the available information remains inconclusive. As noted in the first Framingham analysis, only elderly people consuming vitamin D supplements received a BMD benefit from dairy consumption. This suggests that a more effective strategy for maintaining bone health is to achieve adequate blood vitamin D levels, which are essential for optimal calcium absorption regardless of its source. For most people year round, and virtually everyone at northern latitudes in the winter, this means taking a vitamin D supplement. Adequate vitamin D levels appear to be crucial to any bone health benefit of dairy.

OTHER DIETARY FACTORS AFFECT BONE HEALTH

Milk is just one of many beverages, and these other beverages could play roles in bone health. Turning yet again to an analysis of the Nurses' Health Study by the Harvard Nutrition Department, elevated intakes of soft drinks by post-menopausal women were associated with an increased risk of hip fractures.[218] For women without diabetes, each daily serving of a regular soda (containing sugar and caffeine) conferred an additional 19% risk for hip fracture. For women with diabetes, the increased risk appeared to be even greater. Consumption of diet soda or non-caffeinated soda seemed to be slightly less harmful, but the trend was not significant compared to regular soda. These researchers also examined milk consumption in this group, and found that increased soda consumption was not associated with decreased milk drinking. Thus, the deleterious effect of soda on hip fractures appears to be a direct effect of soda itself, rather than a secondary effect from reduced milk intake. This report is consistent with an earlier study based on the Framingham dataset that indicated a relationship between increased cola consumption and reduced BMD in older women.[219] It is interesting to compare the magnitude of the effect of one soda per day (a 19% increase in hip fractures) versus the 8% fracture reduction for one glass of milk per day seen in the Harvard analysis of the Nurses' Health Study and Health Professionals Follow-up Study. The health-concerned should readily see the message here.

In closing it appears that, in the context of adequate vitamin D and weight-bearing exercise, perhaps dairy calcium does have a significant role in preventing fractures. In the literature just described, chronically low vitamin D levels may have underlain the failure of dairy to protect against fractures in the elderly. Apparently no studies have evaluated a potential protective effect of dairy in the context of adequate vitamin D and sufficient exercise. Certainly no one should assume that dairy intake alone is an insurance against future fractures. Dairy consumption to maintain bone health appears to be a reasonable precaution, although this approach is not really supported by unequivocal science.

DOES GENETICALLY DETERMINED LACTASE NONPERSISTENCE AFFECT BONE HEALTH?

Given the overall emphasis of this book, an obvious question is the impact of genetic nonpersistence (that is, individuals lacking one of the SNPs that confer lactase production into adulthood) on bone health. A large Dutch study determined the status of the -13,910 SNP in about 9200 older men and women who were participants in two long-term studies, the Rotterdam Health Study and the Longitudinal Aging Study Amsterdam.[220] About 30% of this population was homozygous for the -13,910 C genotype, and therefore lactase non-persistent. These non-persistent individuals had slightly lower calcium intake due to decreased consumption of both milk and other dairy products. Despite this, the lactase non-persistent subjects did not suffer a decrease in BMD or an increase in fractures compared to the persistent subjects. Generally the subjects, regardless of lactase status, consumed substantial amounts of calcium, and over half of this intake was from non-dairy sources. In a population that was more calcium deprived, a similar study may have produced different results. Not surprisingly, other studies have yielded differing results, showing lactase non-persistence to be associated with decreased BMD. In a smaller Hungarian study[221] (590 postmenopausal women) non-persistence was associated with significantly decreased BMD in the hip and lumbar spine. Subjects did not report calcium intake, and perhaps these women consumed less overall calcium than did the well-nourished Dutch elders. In addition, the Hungarian study population consisted of women who had been referred to a bone health clinic, raising the possibility of selection bias. In contrast, the Dutch population was randomly selected. Similar to this Hungarian study, a report based on 395 post-menopausal women in Austria also showed an elevated decrease in lumbar spine and hip BMD in non-persistent participants.[222] Overall, these results are conflicting, and the differing results may arise from variables of diet, lifestyle, and genetics in these populations. However, the results of the large Dutch investigation suggest that effects of non-persistence on BMD and fractures are probably minor.

ARE THERE POTENTIALLY HARMFUL EFFECTS OF DAIRY CONSUMPTION?

An earlier section mentioned a Swedish study that reported an increase in overall mortality with increasing milk consumption. A larger meta-analysis did not confirm this, and showed essentially no effects, good or bad, of dairy consumption on risk of stroke, heart disease, or death.[223] This issue is likely to be explored more in the future; many large longitudinal studies that have tracked dairy consumption also contain mortality data (death is an unequivocal endpoint). The literature contains other reports of potentially harmful effects of dairy. The saturated fat in cheeses and non-skim milk has long been a concern, and more recent research has detailed the size of this risk. One large meta-analysis (over 5 million person-years of data) indicated that dairy fat intake was not related to increased risk of cardiovascular disease (CVD) in this large population.[224] That does not mean that consuming dairy fat is benign. In a typical American diet, dairy fat makes up about 5% of total calorie intake. Computer modelling based on these data indicated that replacing this amount of dairy fat with polyunsaturated fats, such as found in canola oil, would produce to a 24% reduction in CVD. In contrast, replacement with fat from red meat would result in a 6% increase in CVD. Overall, despite decades of research the CVD risk of dairy fat is still somewhat unclear. Its effects are likely highly dependent on the total amount consumed as well as the genetics of individual (recall the earlier discussion of the Maasai, who have low cholesterol despite a diet of whole milk). Of course, for someone concerned about dairy fat, there are many fat-free options in fluid milk and yogurt. Hard cheeses are more of a problem, but even here reduced fat forms are often available.

Aside from the well-known issue of dairy fat, there has been speculation that other components of milk, particularly galactose, may also be harmful. Researchers at the University of North Carolina at Chapel Hill found that elevated milk consumption is associated with an increased rate of mental decline in older people.[225] They based this finding on data from the Atherosclerosis Risk in Communities (ARIC) study. ARIC has followed the health of about 16,000 individuals in four dispersed US communities. This study first evaluated subjects at 45-64 years of age, and additional examinations continued over 27 years. Investigators obtained data on a range of lifestyle factors (including diet) during the study, and they performed cognitive assessments over about the last 20 years. The cognitive battery included tests for word recall, vocabulary, and mathematical associations. They used these results to generate an overall score for cognitive decline. This provided an excellent tool to compare lifestyle factors and diet with the inevitable cognitive decline that occurs with aging. The investigators looked at cognitive decline in subjects in four categories of milk intake: (1) almost never, (2) less than one glass per day, (3) one glass per day, and (4) more than one glass per day. There was a significant association between increased milk intake and increased cognitive decline, and over 20 years the group of highest milk consumers suffered about a 10% increase in mental decline compared to those who almost never consumed milk. The two intermediate groups also showed proportional declines in cognitive function. An additional analysis of data for individuals who consumed only skim milk provided similar findings, showing that increased cognitive decline was not due to saturated fat intake.

The authors conjectured that galactose, produced from the intestinal breakdown of lactose, might cause this cognitive decline. The first chapter described the metabolism of galactose and the developmental problems that can occur in rare individuals unable to convert galactose into glucose. In addition, injections of galactose (but not oral intake) are used to cause premature aging and cognitive decline in mouse and rat models. Galactose is able to react with proteins in the body, and the immune system attacks these modified proteins. The resulting inflammatory response may exacerbate cognitive decline.

The reader should view these findings as preliminary, but this topic bears monitoring. A recent French study yielded somewhat similar results, with increased milk intake associated with decreased cognitive performance in older individuals (mean age of 65.5).[226] However, total dairy product consumption (versus just fluid milk) was not associated with cognitive decline in this group. Since non-milk dairy products generally have much lower levels of lactose (and hence galactose) than fluid milk, this hints that galactose intake could underlie the observed cognitive decline. These authors did not compares intake of fat-free and fat-containing milk, so it is not possible to discern any possible separate influence of dairy fat on cognitive decline.

IMPLICATIONS FOR THE LACTOSE INTOLERANT

As noted at the beginning of this chapter, some populations such as traditional Okinawans live long healthy lives without significant dairy consumption. (Note the use of "traditional", more recently obesity has become a problem in Okinawa because of Japanese and Western influences.) The traditional Okinawan lifestyle included a highly varied diet, substantial exercise, and year-round intense sunlight that aided in adequate vitamin D levels. Based on this, it does not appear essential for the lactose intolerant to consume dairy (in the context of a very healthy lifestyle). However, dairy intake may have a number of important roles such as maintaining muscle and achieving adequate vitamin and mineral intake. The role of dairy in bone health is less clear, though the most recent Framingham analysis suggests a fracture-protective benefit of milk intake by the elderly. Concerned individuals should consider the overall nutrient paucity of many contemporary diets in making a decision about the amount of dairy to consume. Dairy non-consumers must be diligent in consuming other calcium-rich foods. Merely following an often typical modern diet that includes a large amount of nutrient-barren junk food will not result in adequate calcium intake. Diets from past millennia may have been richer in calcium and other minerals than are current diets comprising highly processed foods. This processing often strips minerals and other nutrients from foods, and materials that could have been benefited human health instead end up in animal feed or refuse. Dairy intake is not essential to human health, but dairy avoiders must be very diligent in obtaining nutritional adequacy from other sources.

SUMMARY

The role of milk and dairy products in achieving nutritional adequacy is well established. These foods are good sources of protein, minerals, and several vitamins. Some milk proteins are especially valuable in maintaining muscle mass. Despite the positive nutritional impact of dairy, many human populations consume little or no dairy during adulthood but still maintain good overall health.

Some nutritionists have long touted calcium intake as one of the most important benefits of dairy consumption. Dairy intake does appear to have a role in maintaining BMD, and dairy intake during childhood and adolescence helps build overall bone mass, which may have life-long benefits. The role of adult dairy intake in preventing fractures, particularly debilitating hip fractures, is less clear and any benefit may be relatively minor. For adults the bone health effect of dairy is probably just one factor in a complex equation that involves vitamin D intake, amount of weight-bearing exercise, and other lifestyle factors such as smoking behavior and soda intake. As is the case for most health issues, genetics and even epigenetics probably play a major role.

Some reports have associated increased dairy consumption with CVD, cognitive decline, and increased mortality. The CVD risk can be minimized by reducing dairy fat consumption. The reports of cognitive decline and mortality are concerning, but these reports are few in number and additional confirmatory studies are needed.

14 WHAT DOES THE FUTURE HOLD?

Lactose intolerance appears to be a simple physiological problem caused by childhood loss of a single enzyme in the intestinal villi. This simplicity suggests that novel interventions could be used to mimic the lactose tolerant state, providing a benefit to many sufferers. The discussion of lactase dietary supplements in Chapter 11 noted some deficiencies of current products, including the sensitivity of this lactase to stomach proteases and acidity, as well as its short residence time in the small intestine. A significant improvement may lie in an enzyme that could survive passage through the stomach to reach the small intestine, and then adhere to the lining of the small intestine. This would mimic the function of the natural human lactase. A few academic research groups have focused on this area of lactase improvement, and they have achieved some successes in solving these challenges. Although none of these innovations has yet led to a commercial product, this work indicates that major improvements are feasible. This brief chapter examines these efforts.

MODIFYING LACTASE TO INCREASE IN VIVO EFFICACY

Developing an enzyme that would adhere to the intestine might seem straightforward, compared to the highly sophisticated medical interventions that are common today. However, this approach faces multiple challenges. First, the enzyme must survive a gauntlet of acid attack and protein destroying enzymes in the stomach before entering the more benign environment of the small intestine.

Second, some binding mechanism must attach the enzyme to the surface of the small intestine, preventing its otherwise rapid passage to the colon. A technology imitating a lactose tolerant person's digestion must deal with these two challenges.

Researchers at the University of Limerick in Ireland pursued a sustained release approach.[227] (Ireland is a somewhat unexpected place for such work since it has the world's highest rate of adult lactase persistence.) Enzyme companies have commercialized two types of lactase. One is a yeast (*Kluyveromyces*) enzyme that is most active at around neutral pH (7.0), and is very sensitive to inactivation by stomach acid. Its primary use is the production of lactose-free milk because of this sensitivity to gastric attack. The second, produced by various strains of a filamentous fungus (*Aspergillus*), is most active at an acidic pH and less sensitive to stomach acid inactivation. Dietary supplements typically use lactase derived from *Aspergillus*. The Irish combined these two enzymes in a novel delivery form that releases the *Aspergillus* enzyme into the stomach, where it is most active, and delays the release of the yeast enzyme until it reaches the more benign environment of the intestine. To do this, they placed the yeast enzyme inside of a small capsule, which they then enterically coated. (An enteric coating remains intact in the acid conditions of the stomach, but quickly breaks down in the neutral intestine.) They packed this small capsule along with *Aspergillus* lactase powder inside a larger, non-enteric coated capsule.

The researchers intended this non-coated capsule to release an initial burst of fungal lactase after it was swallowed and entered the stomach. Following this, a second burst of lactase would be released after the surviving enteric coated capsule reached the intestine and dissolved. They tested this novel capsule inside a capsule prototype in vitro, and it behaved just as the inventors had intended. However, they apparently did not test this interesting prototype in humans. One biological challenge of this approach is that the timing of the passage of the enteric capsule into the intestine could be erratic, and might not occur until almost all lactose from dairy intake had already passed through the upper intestine. The stomach tends to retain large particulates like this coated capsule during digestion, so that the stomach's grinding action has a longer time to try to break them into smaller more digestible particles. Finally, the stomach dumps remaining large food particles into the intestine at the end of a meal's digestion in a cleansing wave.[228] One approach to this problem not considered by the authors would be to incorporate the yeast enzyme into tiny enteric coated particles. If sufficiently small, perhaps a few hundred microns in diameter, the stomach would gradually release these enzyme particles into the intestine throughout the digestion of a meal. This would provide some level of lactase in the intestine at all times during digestion. Although this approach does potentially extend the contact time between enzyme and lactose because of the relatively long transit time through the small intestine, it does not provide a mechanism for attaching the enzyme to the GI tract surface. However, the use of such enteric coatings at least permits lactase to survive passage through the stomach and work in the small intestine. The yeast lactase should be quite effective in this environment, with improved efficacy compared to current products.

In a separate effort to improve lactase efficacy, the researchers in Limerick modified the enzyme itself.[229] Polyethylene glycols (PEG) are highly water soluble polymers with many industrial uses, including food applications. Some biotechnology applications involve chemically linking PEG to protein drugs. These PEGylated proteins possess novel properties compared to the original proteins, including improved stability and resistance to protein-degrading enzymes. The PEG on the surface of the protein apparently acts as a shield against attack by these proteases. This Irish group coupled PEG to an acid-active *Aspergillus* lactase and compared the properties of this PEGylated lactase to untreated enzyme. In contrast to this control, PEGylated lactase showed improved activity at acid pH in the range of 2.5 to 4.5. However, a pH of 1.5 totally inactivated both PEGylated and control enzymes. This pH is very acidic but easily attained in the stomach after meals. The PEGylated lactase was also less prone to inactivation by pancreatin, a mixture of protease-containing enzymes that the pancreas releases into the small intestine during digestion. This work demonstrated that a simple chemical modification of lactase could improve its properties, at least as assessed in the laboratory. The Irish researchers apparently did not test this PEGylated lactase in people. It is unclear if commercialization of this approach could be justified in light of the likely high development costs. Although food regulations permit use of some types of PEG, the chemicals these scientists used to couple PEG to lactase are not approved for food use. An innovator would have to pursue complex toxicology testing and obtain regulatory approvals in order to bring this modified enzyme to the market. As with the other attempts to improve efficacy, a deficiency of this approach is that it does not result in an enzyme that binds to the intestine.

APPLICATIONS OF NANOTECHNOLOGY

A different approach sought to engineer a lactase that could attach to the surface of the small intestine, mimicking the human enzyme. A research group in Yantai, China, applied the rapidly advancing field of nanotechnology, which exploits the unique properties of extremely small particles (nanoparticles). They developed lactase nanoparticles that appear to be capable of attaching to the intestine and remaining in place for considerable time.[230]

In the first step of their complex process, they entrapped yeast lactase inside of porous particles of poly(lactic acid), or PLA, which is a food-grade polymer. These PLA particles are sufficiently permeable so that small molecules like lactose can readily diffuse into them. The entrapped lactase cleaves the lactose, and the simple sugars diffuse out of the particles. The lactase protein itself is too large to diffuse out of the particles, and protein-destroying digestive enzymes are too large to penetrate into the particles. The lactase is essentially inside a protective cage that blocks protease attack. These scientists then applied a coating to the PLA particles that caused them to become mucoadhesive; that is, they attach to the mucus coating of the intestinal surface. This coating was a combination of wheat germ agglutinin and soluble chitosan. Wheat germ agglutinin is a protein extracted from wheat kernels. It has the interesting property of binding to sialic acid, which is a major component of the polymers that form mucus. Chitosan is a material that forms the hard outer shells of crustaceans such as lobsters and shrimp. After conversion to a soluble form, it serves a role in stabilizing the nanoparticles, and helps them remain suspended as individual particles rather than clumping together, which is a common problem in nanotechnology.

A series of test tube and animal experiments demonstrated the potential benefits of these lactase nanoparticles. When incubated in a solution of pancreatin, the nanoparticles strongly protected lactase from degradation. In contrast, pancreatin quickly inactivated unencapsulated lactase. They also compared the rates of breakdown of lactose by lactase nanoparticles and lactase in solution. Based on the amount of enzyme, the rate of breakdown by the nanoparticles was somewhat slower than the lactose hydrolysis rate by lactase in solution. This is to be expected, because lactose has to diffuse into the nanoparticles, which slows the reaction. However, improved stability of the lactase inside nanoparticles more than compensated for this slight decrease in activity. Finally, the investigators orally gavaged nanoparticles into the stomachs of rats, and measured the amount of nanoparticles remaining in the rat intestines 24 hours later. The particles had an intestinal half-life (the time when one-half the original particles remain) of about seven hours. Furthermore, a substantial portion of the particles remained in the intestine at 24 hours after dosing.

These results are of course very preliminary, and await confirmation in human trials. In addition, this approach does not appear to protect lactase from damage in the stomach. Likely an enteric coating to provide safe passage through the stomach would solve this problem. Overall, this pioneering research suggests that a tablet of nanoparticle lactase could be taken once a day, with some amount of functional enzyme remaining in the intestine for many hours. This could allow a consumer to swallow a lactase tablet at breakfast. It would continue to work day, eliminating the need to take lactase just before consuming dairy. With this breakthrough product, the physiology of lactose-intolerant people would begin to resemble that of the lactose tolerant.

Converting this prototype into a product on the store shelf would require enormous work. Because of the chemicals used in the production of these nanoparticles, it is possible that the final product would be a prescription drug, rather than a supplement conveniently available to all consumers. Regardless, this approach requires very extensive safety testing in animals and humans. In addition, product price could be of concern since the innovator would want to recoup the extensive development and manufacturing costs. Finally, and possibly the greatest cause of concern, lies in the potential toxicity of the nanoparticles themselves. The Chinese researchers reported that some nanoparticles were absorbed through the rats' intestines, and ended up in the blood, liver, spleen, and kidneys. The potential toxicity of oral exposure to nanoparticles has raised widespread concerns.[231] Of particular concern is the systemic absorption of nanoparticles that do not quickly breakdown, which potentially could result in their accumulation to toxic levels in some tissues. The overall evaluation of safety of the lactase nanoparticles would perhaps be the greatest barrier to getting this innovation into the hands of consumers. However, given the rapid advances in biotechnology, a new long-acting lactase may eventually become available, providing lactose intolerant consumers with convenience and confidence.

15 EPILOGUE

We have explored the complex story of dairy domestication and its impact on human genetics and culture. The appearance of lactase persistence is just one recent example of how our genetics is adapting to cultural changes.

At one time, lactose intolerance posed a barrier to dairy consumption for many people. However, the development of lactase supplements and lactose-free dairy products has ameliorated this situation. In addition, consumption of appropriate probiotics or prebiotics may control symptoms of intolerance in some individuals.

Milk has often been touted as the "perfect food," and marketing propaganda from various sources has conspired to make non-dairy consumers feel inadequate or even guilty. However, the consumption of dairy has appeared very late in human evolution, and there is certainly no necessity to consume dairy in order to enjoy good health. In fact, many contemporary societies consume little or no dairy after childhood. This group includes some of the world's healthiest societies, measured in terms of morbidity and mortality. However, the diets of many people in "advanced" countries are depleted in key nutrients such as calcium, and the dairy avoider must be very diligent in achieving nutritional adequacy from a range of other foods. Also, these "modern" people are often lacking the intense and frequent exercise that helps maintain bone and muscle mass in aging, and the nutrients in dairy products may somewhat ameliorate these culture-induced health problems.

The revolutions in biotechnology and genetic engineering open the door to new options for dealing with lactose intolerance. However, commercialization of these innovations would involve large safety hurdles, and it is unclear if any of these will be commercialized in the upcoming decades.

ABOUT THE AUTHOR

Thomas Sox has had a long fascination with lactose intolerance, despite being definitely lactose tolerant. For over 20 years as a scientist with a major health care company, he investigated technology for treating lactose intolerance. He keenly followed the rapid changes in our knowledge of the development of lactose tolerance and its implications. This book captures his knowledge and insights from this long-term endeavor. It narrates a complex story of how domestication of dairy animals altered both human evolution and culture.

Dr. Sox received a BA in Zoology from Duke University, a PhD in Microbiology and Immunology from the University of North Carolina at Chapel Hill, and a JD from Temple University. For most of his career, he conducted research in various areas of healthcare for Procter and Gamble and Johnson and Johnson. He currently consults for the healthcare and nutrition industries, and is a member of the Pennsylvania and US Patent bars. A love of biology developed at an early age has led to his life-long fascination with bacteria, bees, plants, and almost any other aspect of biological sciences.

INDEX

REFERENCES

[1] Canadian Dairy Information Centre, accessed 10/23/2017. Dairy.info.gc.ca.

[2] Messer, M, and KR Kerry. "Milk Carbohydrates of the Echidna and the Platypus." *Science* 180 (1973): 201-203.

[3] Coelho, AL, ME Rubio-Gozalbo, JB Viente, JB, and I Rivera. "Sweet and Sour: an Update on Classical Galactosemia." *J Inherited Metabolic Diseases* 40 (2017): 325-342.

[4] Hill, P, Schieber, A, Yildirin, C, Arnold, et al. "Detection of Phloridzin in Strawberries (Fragaria x anassa Duch.) by HPLC-PDA-MS/MS and NMR Spectroscopy." *Agricultural and Food Chemistry* 51 (2003): 2896-2899.

[5] Lomer, MCE, GC Parkes, and JD Sanderson. "Review Article: Lactose Intolerance in Clinical Practice – Myths and Realities." *Alimentary Pharmacology and Therapeutics* 27 (2008): 93-103.

[6] Jacob, F. "The Birth of the Operon." *Science* 332 (2011): 767.

[7] Brüssow, Harald. pp. 6-10, Chapter 1, "A Nutritional Conditio Humana", in *The Quest for Food: A Natural History of Eating*, Springer, New York, 2007. ISBN-10: 0-387-30334-0.

[8] Marciniak, A. "The Secondary Products Revolution: Empirical Evidence and Its Current Zooarcheological Critique." *J World Prehistory* 24 (2011): 117-130.

[9] Scott, JC. *Against the Grain – A Deep History of the Earliest States*. Yale University Press, 2017.

[10] Macintosh, AA, R Pinhasi, and JT Stock. "Early Life Conditions and Physiological Stress Following the Transition to Farming in Central/Southeast Europe: Skeletal Growth Impairment and 6000 Years of Gradual Recovery." *PLoS ONE* 11(2) (2016): e148468. Doi:10.1371/journal.pone.0148468.

[11] Lillie, M. "Vedrovice: Demography and Paleopathology in an Early Farming Population." *Anthropolgie* XLV/2-3 (2008): 135-152.

[12] Diamond, J., Chapter 11 "The Lethal Gift of Livestock", p. 207, in *Guns, Germs, and Steel – The Fates of Human Societies*. WW Norton & Company, New York, 1999.

[13] Huyge, D. "Late Paleolithic and Epipaleolithic Rock Art in Egypt: Qurta and El-Hosh." *Archeo-Nil* 19 (2009): 109-120.

[14] Caeser, GJ, Book VI, paragraph XXVIII in *Commentaries on the Gallic War*. Translated by WA McDevitte and WS Bohn, Harper & Brothers, New York, 1869.

[15] Utsonomiya, YT, M Milanesi, ATH Utosonomiya, RBP Torrecilha, et al. "A *PLAG1* Mutation Contributed to Stature Recovery in Modern Cattle." *Scientific Reports* 7 (2017): 17140.

[16] Loftus, RT, DEMacHugh, DG Bradley, PM Sharp, and P Cunningham. "Evidence for Two Independent Domestications of Cattle." *Proc. Natl. Acad. Sci. USA* 91 (1994): 2757-2761.

[17] Hongo, H, J Pearson, J, B Oksuz, and G Ilgezdi. "The Process of Ungulate Domestication at Cayonu, Southeastern Turkey: a Multidisciplinary Approach Focusing on *Bos* sp. and *Cervus elaphus*." *Anthropozoologica*. 44 (2009): 63-78.

[18] Bollongino, R, J Burger, A Powell, M Mashkour, et al. "Modern Taurine Cattle Descended from Small Numbers of Near-Eastern Founders." *Mol Biol Evol* 29 (2012): 2101-2104.

[19] Park, SDE, DA Magee, PA McGettigan, MD Teasdale et al. "Genomic Sequencing of the Extinct Eurasian Wild Aurochs, *Bos primigenius* Illuminates the Phylogeography and Evolution of Cattle." *Genome Biology* 16 (2015): 234 doi:10.1186/s13059-015-0790-2.

[20] Randhawa, IAS, MS Khatkar, PC Thompson, and HW Raadswa. "A Meta-Analysis of Selection Signatures in Cattle." *PLoS One* 11(4) (2016): e0153013. Doi:10.1371/journal.pone.015013.

[21] Fiems, LF. "Double Muscling in Cattle: Genes, Husbandry, Carcasses and Meat." *Animals* 2 (2012): 472-506.

22 Upadhyay, M, VH da Silvia,H-J, Megans, MHPW Visker, et al. "Distribution and Functionality of Copy Number Variation across European Cattle Populations." *Frontiers in Genetics* 8 (2017): article 108, doi:10.3389/fgene.2017.00108.

23 Vigne, J-D, ICarrere, F Briois, and J Guilaine. "The Early Process of Mammal Domestication in the Near East – New Evidence from Pre-Neolithic and Pre-Pottery Neolithic in Cyprus." *Current Anthropology* 52 (suppl 4) (2011): S255-S271.

24Simmons, AH. Chapter 8 "The Earliest Residents of Cyprus, Ecological Pariahs or Harmonious Settlers?" in *The Archeology of Environmental Change, Socionatural Legacies of Degradation and Resilience* (Fisher, CT, Hill, JB, Feinman, GM, eds), The University of Arizona Press, Tucson, 2009.

25 Edwards, CJ, C Ginja,and J Kantanen. "Dual Origins of Dairy Cattle Farming – Evidence from a Comprehensive Survey of European Y-Chromosomal Variation." *PLoS One* 6 (Jan 2001): e15922.

26 Chin, S, B-ZLin, M Baig, B Mitra, et al. "Zebu Cattle are an Exclusive Legacy of the South East Asia Neolithic." *Mol Biol Evol* 27(1) (2010): 1-6.

27 Beja-Pereira, A, D Carameli, C Laluez-Fox, C Vernesi, N Ferrand, et al. "The Origin of European Cattle: Evidence from Modern and Ancient DNA." *Proc. Natl. Acad. Sci. USA* 103 (2006): 8113-8118.

28 Pitt, D, N Servane, EL Nicolazzi, DE MacHugh, et al. "Domestication of Cattle: Two or Three events?" *Evolutionary Applications* 2018;00:1-14. doi.org/10.1111/eva12674.

29 Frisch, W. Der Auerochs: Das europaische Rind, 2010.

30 Anonymous. Tauros Programme, https://www.rewildingeurope.com/tauros-programme, accessed June 30, 2017.

31 Exodus, Chapter 32. Holy Bible, King James Version.

32 Harris, M. Article 34 "India's Sacred Cow" pp. 201-207, in *Anthropology Contemporary Perspectives, Sixth Ed.,* ed by P Whitten and DEK Hunter, Scott Foresman and Company, Glenview IL, 1990.

33 Evershed, RP, S Payne, G Sherratt, MS Copley, J Coolidge, et al. "Earliest Date for Milk Use in the Near East and Southeastern Europe Linked to Cattle Herding." *Nature* 455 (2018): 528-531.

34 Warriner, C, J Hendy, C Speller, E Cappellini, et al. "Direct Evidence of Milk Consumption from Ancient Human Calculus. *Sci. Rep.* 4, 7104; DOI:10:1038/srep07104(2014).

35 Salque, M, PI Bogucki, J Pyzel, I Sobkowiak-Tabaka, R Grygiel, et al. "Earliest Evidence for Cheese Making in the Sixth Millennium BC in Northern Europe. *Nature* 493 (2013): 5322-525.

36 Grygiel, R. *The Neolithic and Early Bronze Age in the Brześć Kujawski and Olsonki Region, Vol. 1,* Konrad Jaździewski Foundation for Archeological Research, Museum of Archeology and Ethnography, Lódź, Poland, 2004.

37 Gerbault, C, C Moret, M Currat, and A Sanchez-Mazas. "Impact of Selection and Demography on the Diffusion of Lactase Persistence." *PLoS ONE* 4(7) (2009): e6369. Doi:10.1371/journal.pone.0006369.

38Hery, F-X, and T Enel. Figure 193 in *Animaux du Nil Animaux de Dieu* , p 158. C-Y Chaudoreille, Edisud, Aix-en-Provence, France, 1993.

39 van Noten, FL., X Misonne, and H Rhotert. "Rock Art of the Jebel Uweinat Libyan Sahara: Contributions by Hans Rhotert and Xavier Misonne." *Akad. Dr.-und Verlag-Anst*, 1978.

40 Phillips, CJC. Chapter 1 "The Development of the World's Cattle Production Systems", p. 3, in *Principles of Cattle Production*, CABI International, Wallingford, UK, 2001.

41Kintisch, E. "The Lost Norse." Science 354 (2016): 696-701.

42 Le Quellec, J-L. "Provoking Lactation by the Insufflation Technique as Documented by Rock Images of the Sahara." *Anthropozoologica* 46 (2011): 65-155.

[43] Werner, Florian.p. 45 in *Cow: A Bovine Biography*, Greystone Books, Vancouver, 2011.

[44] Gandhi, M. p. 242, Chapter 153 "The Rowlatt Bills and My Dilemma," *An Autobiography, The Story of My Experiment with Truth*, Gandhi Book Centre, Bombay, India, 1957.

[45] Government of India. Chap. 3, Section 12, The Prevention of Cruelty to Animals Act 1960, as amended by the Central Act of 1982.

[46] Le Quellec, J-L. "Provoking Lactation by the Insufflation Technique as Documented by the Rock Images of the Sahara." *Anthropozoologica* 46 (2011):65-125.

[47] Food and Agriculture Organization of the United Nations, FAOSTAT, .http://www.fao.org/faostat/en/#search/Cattle, accessed 11/28/2017.

[48] Bar-On, YN, R Phillips, and R Milo. "The Biomass Distribution on Earth." *Proc Natl Acad Sci USA* www.pnas.org/cgi/doi/10.1073/pnas.1711842115 (2018).

[49] van Hooijdonk T, and K Hettinga. "Dairy in a Sustainable Diet: a Question of Balance." *Nutrition Reviews* 73(S1) (2015) :48-54.

[50] Anonymous. Greenhouse Gas Emissions from the Dairy Sector, a Life Cycle Assessment, FAO, Rome, 2010.

[51] Plimmer, RHA. "On the Presence of Lactase in the Intestines of Animals and on the Adaptation of the Intestine to Lactase." *J Physiol* 35 (1906):20-31.

[52] Bayless, TM, and NS Rosensweig. "A Racial Difference in the Incidence of Lactase Deficiency: a Survey of Milk Tolerance and Lactase Deficiency in Healthy Males." *J Amer Med Assoc* 197 (1966): 968-972.

[53] Potter, J, MW Ho, H Bolton, et al. "Human Lactase and the Molecular Basis of lactase Persistence." *Biochemical Genetics* 23 (1985): 423-439.

[54] Johnson, JD. Chapter 2 "The Regional and Ethnic Distribution of Lactose Malabsorption Adaptive and Genetic Hypotheses", p 11-22 in *Lactose Digestion: Clinical and Nutritional Implications* (DM Paige and TM Bayless, eds), The Johns Hopkins University Press, Baltimore, 1981.

[55] Boll, W, P Wagner, and N Mantei. "Structure of the Chromosomal Gene and cDNAs coding for Lactase-Phlorizin Hydrolase in Humans with Adult-Type Hypolactasia or Persistence of Lactase." *Amer J Human Genetics* 48 (1991): 889-902.

[56] Hollox, EJ, M Poulter, M Zvarik, V Ferak, et al. "Lactase Haplotype Diversity in the Old World." *Amer J Human Genetics* 68 (2001): 160-172.

[57] Enattah, NS, T Sabi, E Savilahti, and JD Terwiliger. "Identification of a Variant Associated with Adult-Type Hypolactasia." *Nature Genetics* 30 (2002): 233-237.

[58] The International Hap Map Consortium. "A Second Generation Haplotype Map of over 3.1 Million SNPs." *Nature* 449 (2007): 851-861.

[59] Sharma, A. "Systems Genomics Analysis Centered on Epigenetic Inheritance Supports Development of a Unified Theory of Biology." *J Expt Biol* 218 (2015): 3368-3373.

[60] Labrie, V, OJ Buske, E Oh, R Jeremian, et al." Lactase Non-Persistence Is Directed by DNA Variation-dependent Epigenetic Aging. *Nat Struc Mol Biol* 23 (2016): 566-573.

[61] Liebert, A, BL Jones, ET Danielsen, AK Olsen, et al. "*In Vitro* Functional Analyses of Infrequent Nucleotide Variants in the Lactase Enhancer Reveal Different Molecular Routes to Increase Lactase Promoter Activity and Lactase Persistence." *Ann Human Genetics* 80 (2016): 307-318.

[62] Dzialanski, Z, M Barany, P Engfeldt, P, A Magnuson, et al. "Lactase Persistence versus Lactose Intolerance: Is There an Intermediate Phenotype?" *Clinical Biochemistry* 49 (2016): 248-252.

[63] Hongo, H, J Pearson, B Oksuz, and G Ilgedzi. "The Process of Ungulate Domestication at Cayönü, Southeastern Turkey: A Multidisciplinary Approach Focusing on *Bos* sp and *Cervus elaphus*." *Anthropozoologica* 44(2009):63-78.

64 Itan, Y, A Powell, MA Beauchamp, J Burger, and MG Thomas. "The Origins of Lactase Persistence in Europe." *PLoS Computational Biology* 5 (2009): e1000491.
65 Burger, J, M Kirchner, W Haak, and MG Thomas. "Absence of Lactase-Persistence-Associated Allele in Early Neolithic Europeans." *Proc. Natl. Acad. Sci. USA* 104 (2007): 3736-3741.
66 Segurel, L, Bon, C. "On the Evolution of Lactase Persistence in Humans." *Ann Rev of Genomics and Human Genetics* 18 (2017): 8.1-8.13.
67 Sabeti, PC, SF Schaffner, B Fry, J Lohmueller, et al. "Positive Natural Selection in the Human Lineage." *Science* 312 (2006): 1614-1620.
68 Bersaglieri, T, PC Sabeti, N Patterson, T Vanderploeg, et al." Genetic Signatures of Strong Recent Positive Selection at the Lactase Gene." *Amer J Human Genetics* 74 (2004): 1111-1120.
69 Flatz, G, and HW Rotthauwe. "Lactose Nutrition and Natural Selection." *Lancet* 302 (1073): 76-77.
70 Suarez, FL, D Savaiano, P Arbisi, P, and MD Levitt. "Tolerance to the Daily Ingestion of Two Cups of Milk by Individuals Claiming Lactose Intolerance." *Amer J Clin Nutr* 65 (1997): 1502-1506.
71 Pray, WS. "Lactose Intolerance: the Norm among the World's People." *Amer J Pharma Education* 64 (2000): 205-207.
72 Meyer, C, C Lohr, D Gronenborn, and KW Alt. "The Massacre Mass Grave of Schoneck-Kilianstadten Reveals New Insights into Collective Violence in Early Neolithic Central Europe." *Proc Nat Acad Sci* 112 (2015): 11217-11222.
73Hoang, TT, Y Lei, LE Mitchell, SV Sharma, et al. "Maternal Lactase Polymorphism (rs4988235) Is Associated with Neural Tube Defects in Offspring in the National Birth Defects Prevention Study." *J of Nutrition* 148 (2019):1-0.
74 Edmonds, CA, AS Lillie, and LL Cavalli-Sforza. "Mutations Arising in the Wave Front of an Expanding Population." *Proc Natl Acad Sci USA* 101 (2004): 975-979.
75 Beja-Pereira, A, G Luikar, and PR England. "Gene-Culture Coevolution between Cattle Milk Protein Genes and Human Lactase Genes." *Nature Genetics* 35 (2003): 311-313.
76 Malasse, M, and A Tresset. "Early Weaning of Neolithic Domestic cattle (Bercy, France) Revealed by Intra-Tooth Variation in Nitrogen Isotope *Analysis." J Archaeological Sci* 29 (2002): 853-859.
77 McCullough, JM, KM Heath, and AM Smith. "Hemochromatosis: Niche Construction and the Genetic Domino Effect in the European Neolithic." *Human Biology* 87 (2015): 39-58.
78 Hallberg, L, L Rossander-Hulten, M Brune, and A Gleerup. "Bioavailability in Man of Iron in Human Milk and Cow's Milk in Relation to Their Calcium Contents." *Pediatric Research* 31 (1992): 524-528.
79 Walker, L, P Bathurst, R Richman, T Gjerdrum, et al. "The Causes of Porotic Hyperostosis and Cribra Orbitalia: a Reappraisal of the Iron-deficiency-anemia Hypothesis." *Amer J Clinical Anthropology* 139 (2009): 109-125.
80 Jones, BL, T Oljira, A Liebert, P Zmarz, N Nontalva, et al. "Diversity of Lactase Persistence in African Milk Drinkers." *Human Genet* 134 (2015): 917-925.
81 Torniainen, S, MI Parker, V Holmberg, E Lahtela, et al. "Screening of Variants for Lactase Persistence/Non-persistence in Populations from South Africa and Ghana." *BMC Genetics* 10 (2009): 31, doi:10.1186/1471-2156-10-31.
82 Jakobsson, M, SW Scholz, P Scheet, JR Gibbs, et al. "Genotype, Haplotype, and Copy-Number Variation in Worldwide Human Populations." *Nature* 451 (2008):998-994.
83 Macholdt, E, M Slatkin, B Pakendorf, and M Stoneking. "New Insight into the History of the C-14010 Lactase Persistence Variant in Eastern and Southern Africa." *Amer J Phys Anthropol* 156 (2015): 661-664.

[84] Wagh, K, A Bhatia, G Alexe, A Reddy, et al. "Lactase Persistence and Lipid Pathway Selection in the Maasai." *PLoS One* 7(9) (2012): e44751.

[85] Breton, G, CM Schlebusch, M Lombard, P Sjodin, et al. "Lactase Persistence Alleles Reveal Partial East African Ancestry of Southern African Khloe Pastoralists." *Current Biology* 24 (2014): 852-858.

[86] Ranciaro, A, MC Campbell, JB Hirbo, W-Y Ko, A Froment, et al. "Genetic Origins of Lactase Persistence and the Spread of Pastoralism in Africa." *Amer J Hum Genet* 94 (2014): 496-510.

[87] fao.org/agriculture/dairy-gateway/milk-production/dairy-animals/camels. Accessed 9-14-2017.

[88] Yagul, Y. FAO Animal and Health Paper "Camels and Camel Milk", FAO Corporate Document Repository, Rome, 1982. ISBN 92-5-101169-9

[89] Hill,SC, TR Mohammed, and T Kivisild, T. "Brief Communication: Effect of Nomadic Subsistence Practices on Lactase Persistence Associated Genetic Variation in Kuwait." *Amer J Physical Anthropol* 152 (2013):140-144.

[90] Jones, BL, TO Ragu, TO, A Liebert, P Zmarz, et al. "Diversity of Lactase Persistence Alleles in Ethiopia: Signature of a Soft Selective Sweep." *Amer J Human Genetics* 93 (2103):538-544.

[91] Jones, BL, T Oljira, A Liebert, P Zmarz, et al. "Diversity of Lactase Persistence in African Milk Drinkers." *Human Genetics* 134 (2015): 917-925.

[92] Imtiaz, F, E Savilahti, A Savnesto, K Al-Kahtani, et al. "The T/G Variant Upstream of the Lactose Gene (LCT) Is the Founder Allele of Lactase Persistence in an Urban Saudi Population." *J Medical Genetics* 44 (2007): e89. doi:10.1136/jmg2007.051631.

[93] Babu, J, S Kunar, P Babu, JH Prasad, et al. "Frequency of Lactose Malabsorption among Healthy Southern and Northern Indian Populations by Genetic Analysis and Lactose Hydrogen Breath and Tolerance Tests." *Amer J Clin Nutr* 91 (2010): 140-146.

[94] Heyer, E, A Brazier, L Segurel, T Hegay, et al. "Lactase Persistence in Central Asia: Phenotype, Genotype, and Evolution." *Human Biol* 83 (2011): 379-392.

[95] Ennatah, NS, A Trudeau, V Pimenoff, L Maiuri, et al. "Evidence of Still-Ongoing Convergence Evolution of the Lactase Persistence Allele T -13910 in Humans." *Amer J Human Genetics* 81 (2007): 615-623.

[96] Qiu, Q, L Wang, K Wang, Y Yang, et al. "Yak Whole-Genome Sequencing Reveals Domestication Signatures and Prehistoric Population Expansion." *Nature Communications* 6 (2015): 10283 doi: 10.1038/ncommons10283.

[97] Peng, M-S, J-D He, C-L Chu, C-L, S-F Wu, et al. "Lactase Persistence May Have an Independent Origin in Tibetan Populations from Tibet, China." *J Human Genetics* 57 (2012): 394-397.

[98] Yang, J-F, M Fox, H Chu, X Zheng, X, Y-Q Long, et al. "Four Sample Lactose Hydrogen Breath Test for Diagnosis of Lactose Malabsorption in Irritable Bowel Syndrome Patients with Diarrhea." *World J Gastroenterol* 21 (2015): 7563-7570.

[99] Swallow, DM and JT Troelsen. "Escape from Epigenetic Silencing of Lactase Expression Is Triggered by a Single Nucleotide Change." *Nature Struc Mol Biol* 21 (2016): 505-507.

[100] Perry, GF, NJ Dominy, KG Claw, AS Lee, et al. "Diet and Evolution of Human Amylase Copy Number Variation." *Nature Genetics* 39 (2007): 1256-1260.

[101] Axelsson, E, A Ratnakumar, M-L Arendt, K Maqbool, et al. "The Genomic Signature of Dog Domestication Reveals Adaptation to a Starch-Rich Diet." *Nature* 495 (2013): 360-364.

[102] Arendt, M, KM Cairns, WJO Ballard, P Savolainen, et al. "Diet Adaptation in Dog Reflects Spread of Prehistoric Agriculture." *Heredity* 117 (2016): 301-306.

[103] Carmody, RN, M Danneman, AW Briggs, B Nicket, et al. "Genetic Evidence of Human Adaptation to a Cooked Diet." *Genome Biol Evol* 8 (2016): 1091-1103.

[104] Harvey, CB, Y Wang, LA Hughes, and DM Swallow. "Studies on the Expression of Intestinal Lactase in Different Individuals." *Gut* 36 (1985): 28-33.

[105] Solomons, NW, R Garcia-Ibanez, and FE Viteri. "Hydrogen Breath Test of Lactose Absorption in Adults: The Application of Physiological Doses and Whole Cow's Milk Sources." *Amer J Clin Nutr* 33 (1980): 545-554.

[106] Levitt, MD. "Production and Excretion of Hydrogen Gas in Man." *New England J of Medicine* 281 (1969): 122-127.

[107] Simren, M, and P-O Stotzer. "Use and Abuse of Breath Hydrogen Tests." *Gut* 55 (2006): 297-303.

[108] Solomons, NW, R Garcia-Ibanez, and F Viteri. "Reduced Rate of Breath Hydrogen Excretion with Lactose Tolerance Tests in Young Children Using Whole Milk." *Amer J Clin Nutr* 32 (1979): 783-786.

[109] McKay, LF, MA Eastwood, and WG Brydon. "Methane Excretion in Man – a Study of Breath, Flatus, and Faeces." *Gut* 26 (1985):69-74.

[110] Houben, E, V De Preter, J Billen, M Van Ranst, and K Verbeke. "Additional Value of CH_4 Measurement in a Combined $^{13}C/H_2$ Lactose Malabsorption Test: a Retrospective Analysis." *Nutrients* 7 (2015): 7469-7485.

[111] Krawczyk, M, M Wolska, S Schwartz, G Gruenhage, et al. "Concordance of Genetic and Breath Hydrogen Tests for Lactose Intolerance in a Tertiary Referral Centre." *J Gastroenterol Liver Dis* 17 (2008): 135-139.

[112] Jellema, P, FG Schellevis, DAWM van Der Windt, CMF Kneepkens, et al. "Lactose Malabsorption and Intolerance: a Systematic Review on the Diagnostic Value of Gastrointestinal Symptoms and Self-Reported Milk Intolerance." *Quarterly J Medicine* 103 (2010):555-572.

[113] Mantovani, MP, S Guandalini, P Ecuba, et al. "Lactose Malabsorption in Children with Symptomatic *Giardia Lamblia* Infection: Feasibility of Yogurt Supplementation." *J Pediatric Nutrition and Gastroenterology* 9 (1989): 295-300.

[114] Schirru, E, V Corona, P Usai-Satta, M Scarpa, F Cucca, F, et al. "Decline of Lactase Activity and C/T Variant in Sardinian Children." *J Pediatric Gastroenterology and Nutrition* 45 (2007): 503-506.

[115] Woteki, CE, E Weser, and EA Young. "Lactose Malabsorption in Mexican-American Children." *Amer J Clin Nutr* 29 (1976): 19-24.

[116] Dill, JC, M Levy, RF Wells, and E Weser. "Lactase Deficiency in Mexican American Males." *Amer J Clin Nutr* 25 (1972):869-870.

[117] Garza, C, and NS Scrimshaw. "Relationship of Lactose Intolerance to Milk Intolerance in Young Children." *Amer J Clin Nutr* 29 (1976): 192-196.

[118] Bertron, P, ND Barnard, and M Mills. "Racial Bias in Federal Nutrition Policy, Part 1: The Public Health Implications of Variations in Lactase Persistence." *J Natl Med Assoc* 91 (1999): 151-157.

[119] Paige, DM, TM Bayless, TM, ED Mellitus, and L Davis. "Lactose Malabsorption in Preschool Black Children." *Amer J Clin Nutr* 30 (1977): 1018-1022.

[120] Chiu, CL, NL Hearn, and JM Lind. "Development of a Risk Score for Intestinal Manifestations of Celiac Disease." *Medicine* 95 (2016): 1-6.

[121] Srinivasan, U, E Jones, DG Weir, and C Feighery. "Lactase Enzyme, Detected Immunohistochemically, Is Lost in Active Celiac Disease, But Unaffected by Oats Challenge." *Amer J Gastroenterol* 94 (1999): 2936-2941.

[122] Rezaie, A, M Buresi, A Lembo, H Lin, R McCallum, et al. "Hydrogen and Methane-Based Breath Testing in Gastrointestinal Disorders: The North American Consensus." *Amer J Gastroenterol* 112 (2017): 775-784.

[123] Su, T, S Lai, A Lee, A, X He, S Chen. "Meta-Analysis: Proton Pump Inhibitors Moderately Increase the Risk of Small Intestinal Bacterial Overgrowth." *J Gastroenterol* 53 (2018): 27-36.

[124] Tursi, A, G Brandimarte, GM Giorgetti, and W Elisei. "Transient Lactose Malabsorption in Patients Affected by Symptomatic Uncomplicated Diverticular Disease of the Colon." *Dig Dis Sci* 51 (2006): 461-465.

[125] Ford, AC, BMR Spiegel, NJ Talley, and P Moayyedi. "Small Intestinal Bacterial Overgrowth in Irritable Bowel Syndrome: Systematic Review and Meta-Analysis." *Clin Gastroenterol Hepatol* 7 (2009): 1279-1286.

[126] Lucio, L, G Antonella, and S Mariangela. "High Prevalence of Small Intestinal Bacterial Overgrowth in Lactose Intolerance Patients: Is It a Chicken and Egg Situation?" *British J of Medicine and Medical Res* 4 (2014): 2931-2939.

[127] Majumdar, APN, and MD Basson. Chapter 14 "Effect of Aging on the Gastrointestinal Tract," pp. 405-433, in <u>Physiology of the Gastrointestinal Tract</u>, vol. 1, Fourth Edition (LR Johnson, ed), Elsevier Academic Press, Burlington, MA, 2006.

[128] Di Stefano, M, G Veneto, S Malservisi, A Strocchi, et al. "Lactose Malabsorption and Intolerance in the Elderly." *Scand J Gastroenterol* 36 (2001): 1274-1278.

[129] Suarez, FL, DA Savaiano, and MD Levitt. "A Comparison of Symptoms after the Consumption of Milk or Lactose-Hydrolyzed Milk by People with Self-reported Severe Lactose Intolerance." *New England J Med* 333 (1995): 1-4.

[130] Suarez, FL, D Savaiano, P Arbisi, P, and MD Levitt. "Tolerance to the Daily Ingestion of Two Cups of Milk by Individuals Claiming Lactose Intolerance." *Amer J Clin Nutr* 65 (1997): 1502-1506.

[131] Suchy, FJ, PM Brannon, TO Carpenter, JR Fernandez, et al. National Institute of Health Consensus Development Conference: Lactose Intolerance and Health. *Ann Int Med* 172 (2010): 792-796.

[132] Shaukit, A, MD Levitt, BC Taylor, R MacDonald, et al. "Systematic Review: Effective Management Strategies for Lactose Intolerance." *Ann Int Med* 152 (2010): 797-803.

[133] Kwon, PH, MH Rorick, and NS Scrimshaw. "Comparative Tolerance of Adolescents of Differing Ethnic Backgrounds to Lactose-containing and Lactose-free Dairy Products. II. Improvement of a Double-Blind Test." *Amer J Clin Nutr* 33 (1980): 22-26.

[134] Jones, DV, MC Latham, FW Kosikowski, and G Woodward. "Symptom Response to Lactose-Reduced Milk in Lactose-Intolerant Adults." *Amer J Clin Nutr* 29 (1976): 633-638.

[135] Cavalli-Sforza, LT, and A Strata. "Double-Blind Study on the Tolerance of Four Types of Milk in Lactose Malabsorbers and Absorbers." *Human Nutr Clin Nutr* 41 (1987): 19-30.

[136] Lybeck-Sorensen, K, MV Meersohn, J Sonne, L Larsen, D Edelstein, et al. "A new Type of Low-Lactose Milk. Tolerance by Lactose Malabsorbers and Evaluation of Protein Nutritional Value." *Scand J Gastroenterol* 18 (1983): 1063-1068.

[137] Johnson, AO, JG Semenya, MJ Buchowski, CO Enwonwu, et al. "Correlation of Lactose Maldigestion, Lactose Intolerance and Milk Intolerance." *Amer J Clin Nutr* 57(1993): 399-401.

[138] Haverberg, L, P Kwon, NS Scrimshaw. "Comparative Tolerance of Adolescents of Differing Ethnic Backgrounds to Lactose-Containing and Lactose-Free Dairy Products. I. Initial Experience with a Double-blind Procedure." *Amer J Clin Nutr* 33 (1980): 17-21.

[139] Vonk, RJ, MG Priebe, HA Koetse, F Stellard, et al. "Lactose Intolerance: Analysis of Underlying Factors." *Eur J Clin Invest* 33 (2003): 70-75.

[140] Sterchi, EE, PR Mills, JAM Fransen, H-P Hauri, et al. "Biogenesis of Intestinal Lactase-Phlorizin Hydrolase in Adults with Lactose Intolerance." *Clin Invest* 86 (1990): 1329-1377.

[141] Harvey, CB, Y Wang, LA Hughes, DM Swallow, et al. "Studies on the Expression of Individual Lactase in Different Individuals." *Gut* 36 (1995): 28-33.

142 He, T, K Venema, MG Priebe, et al. "The Role of Colonic Metabolism in Lactose Intolerance." *Eur J Clin Invest* 38 (2008): 541-547.
143 Hertzler, SR, and DA Savaiano. "Colonic Adaptation to Daily Lactose Feeding in Lactose Maldigesters Reduces Lactose Intolerance." *Amer J Clin Nutr* 64 (1996): 232-236.
144 Briet, F, P Pochart, P Marteau, B Flourie, et al. "Improved Clinical Tolerance to Chronic Lactose Ingestion in Subjects with Lactose Intolerance: a Placebo Effect?" *Gut* 41 (1997): 632-635.
145 Rajilic-Stojanovic, M and WM de Vos. "The First 1000 Cultured Species of the Human Gastrointestinal Microbiota." *FEMS Microbiology Reviews* 38 (2014): 996-1047.
146 O'Hara, AM, and F. Shanahan. "The Gut Flora as a Forgotten Organ." *EMBO Reports* 7 (2006): 688-693.
147 Ojetti, V, G Gigante, M Gabrielli, ME Ainora, et al. "The Effect of Oral Supplementation with *Lactobacillus reuteri* or Tilactase in Intolerant Patients: Randomized Trial." *Eur Rev Med and Pharmacol Sci* 14 (2010): 163-170.
148 He, T, MG Priebe, Y Zhong, Y, and C Huang. "Effects of Yogurt and Bifidobacterium Supplementation on the Colonic Microbiota of Lactose-Intolerant Subjects." *J. Applied Bacteriology* 104 (2008): 595-604.
149 Almeida, CC,SLS Lorena, DR Pavan, HMI Akasaka, et al. "Beneficial Effects of Long-Term Consumption of a Probiotic Combination of *Lactobacillus breve* Shirota and *Bifidobacterium breve* Yakult May Persist after Suspension of Therapy in Lactose-intolerant Patients." *Nutr in Clin Pract* 27 (2012): 247-261.
150 Levri, KM, K Ketvertis, M Deramo, JH Merenstein, et al. "Do Probiotics Reduce Adult Lactose Intolerance? A Systematic Review." *J Fam Prac* 54 (2005): 613-620.
151 Rizkalla, SW, J Luo, M Kabir, A Chevalier, et al. "Chronic Consumption of Fresh but Not Heated Yogurt Improves Breath-hydrogen Status and Short-Chain Fatty Acid Profiles: a Controlled Study in Healthy Men with or without Lactose Maldigestion." *Amer J Clin Nutr* 72 (2002): 1474-1479.
152 Martini, MC, EC Lerebours, W-J Lin, SK Harlander, et al. "Strains and Species of Lactic Acid Bacteria in Fermented Milks (Yogurts): Effect on In Vivo Lactose Digestion." *Amer J Clin Nutr* 54 (1991): 1041-1046.
153 McDonough, FE, AD Hitchins, NP Wong, P Wells, et al. "Modification of Sweet Acidophilus Milk to Improve Utilization by Lactose-Intolerant Persons." *Amer J Clin Nutr* 45 (1987): 570-574.
154 Neale, G. "The Diagnosis, Incidence, and Significance of Disaccharidase Deficiency in Adults." *Proc Roy Soc Med* 61 (1968): 1099-1102.
155 Plimmers, RHA. "On the Presence of Lactase in the Intestines of Animals and on the Adaptation of the Intestine to Lactose." *J. Physiology* 35 (1906): 20-31.
156 Dahlqvist, A, JB Hammond, RK Crane, et al. "Intestinal Lactase Deficiency and Lactose Intolerance in Adults: Preliminary Report." *Gastroenterology* 45 (1963):488-491.
157 Dahlqvist, A. "Specificity of the Human Intestinal Disaccharidases and Implications for Hereditary Disaccharide Intolerance." *J Clin Invest* 41 (1962): 463-470.
158 Cuatrecasas, P, DH Lockwood, and JR Caldwell. "Lactase Deficiency in the Adult." *Lancet* 1 (Jan 2) (1965): 14-18.
159 Bayless, TM, and NS Rosensweig. "A Survey of Milk Intolerance and Lactase Deficiency in Healthy Adult Males." *J Amer Medical Assoc* 197 (1966): 138-142.
160Bayless, TM, E Brown, and DM Paige. "Lactase Non-Persistence and Persistence." *Curr Gastroenterol Rep* 19 (2017): 23 doi/org/10.1007/s11894.
161 Huang, S-S, and TM Bayless. "Milk and Lactose Intolerance in Healthy Orientals." *Science* 160 (1968): 83-84.

[162] Bayless, TM, and S-S Huang. "Inadequate Intestinal Digestion of Lactase." *Amer J Clin Nutr* 22 (1969): 250-256.

[163] Mitchell, JD, J Brand, and J Halbisch. "Weight-Gain Inhibition by Lactose in Australian Aboriginal Children." *Lancet* (May 3) (1977): 500-502.

[164] Anonymous. "Lactose, Milk Intolerance, and Feeding Programs." *J Amer Dietetic Assoc* 61 (1972): 241-242.

[165] *Feeding the Crisis: US Food Aid and Farm Policy in Central America*. R. Garst and T Barry, Univ of Nebraska Press, Lincoln, NE, 1990, Note 49, p. 223.

[166] *Feeding the Crisis: US Food Aid and Farm Policy in Central America*. R. Garst and T Barry, Univ of Nebraska Press, Lincoln, NE, 1990, Chapter 7: Food for War, p. 163.

[167] Holsinger, VH. "A Study of the Rehydration Properties of a Milk Analogue Containing Soy Products and Cheese Whey. PhD Dissertation." The Ohio State University, 1980. University Microfilms, Ann Arbor, MI.

[168] Alan Kligerman, personal communication, May, 2017.

[169] "In the Matter of California Milk Producers Board, et al." Docket 8988, 94 FTC 558 (1979).

[170] Clayton, BE, AB Arthur, and DEM Francis. "Early Dietary Management of Sugar Intolerance in Infancy." *Brit Med J* 17 September 1966, 679-682.

[171] Paige, DM, TM Bayless, S-S Huang, and R Wexler. "Lactose Hydrolyzed Milk." *Amer J Clin Nutr* 28 (1975): 818-822.

[172] Turner, SJ, T Daly, JA Hourigan, et al. "Utilization of Low-lactase Milk." *Amer J Clin Nutr* 29 (1976): 739-744.

[173] Jones, DV, MC Latham, FV Kosikowski, et al. "Symptom Response to Lactose-Reduced Milk in Lactose-Intolerant Adults." *Amer J Clin Nutr* 29 (1976): 633-638.

[174] Kligerman, AE, Chapter 24, "Development of Lactose-Reduced Milk Products," pp. 252-256, in <u>Lactose Digestion Clinical and Nutritional Implications</u>, Paige, DM, and Bayless, TM, eds., The Johns Hopkins University Press, Baltimore, MD, 1981.

[175] Solomons, NW, A-M Guerrero, and B Torun. "Dietary Manipulation of Postprandial Colonic Lactose Fermentation: II. Addition of Exogenous, Microbial Beta-galactosidases at Mealtime." *Amer J Clin Nutr* 41 (1985): 209-221.

[176] Rosado, JL, NW Solomons, R Lisker, and H Bourges. "Enzyme Replacement Therapy for Primary Adult Lactase Deficiency: Efficient Reduction of Lactose Malabsorption and Milk Intolerance by Direct Addition of Beta-Galactosidase to Milk at Mealtime." *Gastroenterology* 87 (1984): 1072-1082.

[177] Barillas, C, and NW Solomons. "Effective Reduction of Lactose Maldigestion in Preschool Children by Direct Addition of Beta-Galactosidases to Milk at Mealtime." *Pediatrics* 79 (1987): 766-772.

[178] Solomons, NW, A-M Guerrero, and B Tourin. "Effective In Vivo Hydrolysis of Milk Lactose by Beta-Galactosidases in the Presence of Solid Foods." *Amer J Clin Nutr* 41 (1985): 222-227.

[179] Medow, MS. "Beta-Galactosidase Tablets in the Treatment of Lactose Intolerance in Pediatrics." *Amer J Diseases of Children* 144 (1990): 1261-1264.

[180] Dekker, PJT, D Koenders, and MJ Bruins. "Lactose-Free Dairy Products: Market Developments, Production, Nutrition and Health Benefits." Nutrients 11 (2019) doi: 10.3390/nu11030551.

[181] Gao, K-P, T Mitsui, K Fujiki, H Ishiguro, et al. "Effect of Lactase Preparations in Asymptomatic Individuals with Lactase Deficiency – Gastric Digestion of Lactose and Breath Hydrogen Analysis." *Nagoya J Medical Sciences* 65 (2002): 21-28.

[182] Savaiano, DA, JA Ritter, TR Klaenhammer, GM James, et al. "Improving Lactose Digestion and Symptoms of Lactose Intolerance with a Novel Galacto-Oligosaccharide (RP-G28): a

Randomized Double-blind Clinical Trial." *Nutrition J* 12 (2013): 160-168.

[183] Azcarate-Peril, MA, JA Ritter, AJ, D Savaiano, et al. "Impact of Short-chain Galactooligosaccharides on the Gut Microbiome of Lactose-Intolerant Individuals." *Proc Nat Acad Sci USA* 2017 Jan 17; E367-E375. Doi:10/1073/pnas.1606722113.
[184] Konturek, PC, T Brozozowski, and SJ Konturek. "Stress and the Gut: Pathophysiology, Clinical Consequences, Diagnostic Approach and Treatment Options." *J Physiol Pharmacol* 62 (2011): 591-599.
[185] Mayer, EA, and K Tillisch. "The Brain-Gut Axis in Abdominal Pain Syndromes." *Ann Rev Med* 62 (2011): 381-396.
[186] Gaylord, SA, OS Palsson, EL Garland, et al. "Mindfulness Training Reduces the Severity of Irritable Bowel Syndrome in Women: Results of a Randomized Controlled Trial." *Amer J Gastroenterology* 106 (2011): 1678-1688.
[187] Lackner, JM, GD Gudleski, C-X Ma, et al. "Fear of GI Symptoms Has an Important Impact on Quality of Life in Patients with Moderate-to-Severe IBS." *Amer J Gastroenterol* 109 (2014): 1815-1823.
[188] Lackner, JM. <u>Controlling IBS the Drug-Free Way</u>. Stewart, Tabor & Chang. New York, 2007.
[189] Bharwani, A, A Mian, M Firoz, et al. "Structural and Functional Consequences of Chronic Psychosocial Stress on the Microbiota of the Host." *Psychoneuroendocrinology* 63 (2016): 217-227.
[190] Cenit, MC, Y Sanz, and P Codoner-Franch. "Influence of Gut Microbiota on Neuropsychiatric Disorders." *World J Gastroenterology* 14 (2017): 5486-5498.
[191] Bercik, P, AJ Park, D Sinclair, A Khoshdel, et al. "The Anxiolytic Effect of *Bifidobacterium longum* NCC3001 Involves Vagal Pathways for Gut-Brain Communication." *Neurogastroenterology Motility* 23 (2011): 1132-1140.
[192] Kelly, JR, Y Borre, C O'Brien, et al. "Transferring the Blues: Depression-Associated Gut Microbiota Induces Neurobehavioural Changes in the Rat." *J Psychiatric Res* 82 (2016): 109-118.
[193] Tillisch, K, J Labus, L Kilpatrick, et al. "Consumption of Fermented Milk Product with Probiotic Modulates Brain Activity." *Gastroenterology* 144 (2013): 1394-1401.
[194] Schmidt, K, PJ Cowen, C Harmer, et al. "Prebiotic Intake Reduces the Waking Cortisol Response and Alters Emotional Bias in Healthy Volunteers." *Psychopharmacology* 232 (2015): 1793-1801.
[195] Wilcox, DC, G Scapagnin, and BJ Wlicox. "Healthy Aging Diets Other Than the Mediterranean: A Focus on the Okinawan Diet." *Mech Aging Dev* 136-137 (2014): 148-162.
[196] Deer, RR, and E Volpi. "Protein Intake and Muscle Function in Older Adults". *Curr Opin Clin Nutr Metab Care* 18 (2015): 248-253.
[197] Morley, JE, B Vellas, G Abellan van Kan, SD Anker, et al. "Frailty Consensus: A Call to Action," *J Amer Med Dir Assoc* 14 (2013): 392-397.
[198] Borack, MS, and E Volpi. "Efficacy and Safety of Leucine Supplementation in the Elderly." *J Nutr* 146 (2016): 2625s-2629s.
[199] Lana, A, F Rodriguez-Artalejo, E López-Garcia. "Dairy Consumption and Risk of Frailty in Older Adults: a Prospective Cohort Study." *J Amer Geriatr Soc.* 63 (2010): 1852-1860.
[200] Bradlee, ML, J Mustafa, MR Singer, and LL Moore. "High-Protein Foods and Physical Activity Protect Against Age-Related Muscle Loss and Function Decine. *J Geronotol A Biol Sci Med Sci* 73(2018) :88-94.
[201] Coelho-Júnior, HJ, L Milano-Teixiera, B Rogriguez, et al. "Relative Protein Intake and Physical Function in Older Adults: A Systematic Review and Meta-Analysis of Observational Studies." *Nutrients* 10 (2018). doi:10.3390/nu10091334.

[202]Bauer, J, G Biolo, T Cederholm, M Ceasari, et al. "Evidence-Based Recommendations for Optimal Dietary Protein Intake in Older People: A Position Paper from the PROT-AGE Study Group." *J American Medical Directors Assoc* 14 (2013): 542-599.

[203] Martin, WF, LE Armstrong, and NR Rodriguez. "Dietary Protein Intake and Renal Function." *Nutrition and Metabolism* 2 (2005):25-33. doi:10.1186/1743-7075-2-25.

[204] Weaver, CM. "How Sound Is the Science behind the Dietary Reasons for Dairy?" *Amer J Clin Nutr* 99 (suppl) (2014): 1217S-1222S.

[205] Caroli, A, A Poli, D Ricotta, G Banfi, and D Cocchi. "Invited Review: Dairy Intake and Bone Health: a Viewpoint on the State of the Art." *J Dairy Sci* 94 (2011): 5249-5262.

[206] Weaver, CM, CM Gordon, KF Janz, HJ Kalkwarf, et al. "The National Osteoporosis Foundation's Position Statement on Peak Bone Mass Development and Lifestyle Factors: a Systematic Review and Implementation Recommendations." *Osteoporosis Intl* 27 (2016): 1281-1386.

[207] Salari, P, and M Abdollahi. "The Influence of Pregnancy and Lactation on Bone Health: a Systematic Review." *J Family Reproductive Health* 8 (2014): 135-148.

[208] Crandall, CJ, J Lin, J, Cauley, PA Newcomb, et al. "Association of Parity, Breastfeeding, and Fractures in the Women's Health Observational Study." *Obstet Gynecol* 130 (2017)): 171-180.

[209] Biver, E, C Durosier-Izart, F Merminod, T Chevalley, et al. "Fermented Dairy Products Consumption Is Associated with Attenuated Cortical Bone Loss Independently of Total Calcium, Protein, and Energy Intakes in Healthy Postmenopausal Women." *Osteoporosis Intl* doi.org/10.1007/s00198-018-4535-4 (2018).

[210] Sahni, KM Mangano, DP Kiel, KL Tucker, and MT Hannan, MT. "Dairy Intake Is Protective against Bone Loss in Older Vitamin D Supplement Users: the Framingham Study." *J Nutritional Epidemiology* 147 (2017): 645-652.

[211] Feskanich, D, WC Willett, MJ Stampfer, and GA Colditz. "Milk, Dietary Calcium, and Bone Fractures in Women: a 12-Year Prospective Study." *Amer J Public Health* 87 (1997): 992-997.

[212] Feskanich, D, HA Bischoff-Ferrari, L Frazier, L, and WC Willett. "Milk Consumption during Teenage Years and Risk of Hip Fractures in Older Adults." *J Amer Med Assoc Pediatrics* 168 (2014): 54-60.

[213] Michaelsson, A Wolk, S Langenskiold, S Basu, et al. "Milk Intake and Risk of Mortality and Fractures in Women and Men: Cohort Studies." *Brit Med J* 349 (2014): g6015 doi: 10.1136/bmj.g6015.

[214] Larsson, SC, A Crippa, N Orsini, A Wolk, and K Michaelsson. "Milk Consumption and Mortality from All Causes, Cardiovascular Disease, and Cancer: a Systematic Review and Meta-analysis." *Nutrients* 7 (2015): 7749-7763.

[215] Bischoff-Ferrari, HA, B Dawson-Hughes, JA Baron, EJ Orav, et al. "Milk Intake and Risk of Hip Fracture in Men and Women: a Meta-Analysis of Prospective Cohort Studies." *J Bone Mineral Res* 26 (2011): 833-891.

[216] Sahni, S, KM Mangano, KL Tucker, DP Kiel, et al. "Protective Association of Milk Intake on the Risk of Hip Fracture: Results from the Framingham Original Cohort." *J Bone Mineral Res* 29 (2014): 1756-1762.

[217] Feskanich, D, HE Meyer, TT Fung, HA Bischoff-Ferrari, and WC Willett. "Milk and Other Dairy Foods and Risk of Hip Fractures in Men and Women." *Osteoporosis Intl* 29 (2018): 385-396.

[218] Fung, TT, MH Arasaratnam, F Grodstein, J Katz, et al. "Soda Consumption and Risk of Hip Fractures in Postmenopausal Women in the Nurses' Health Study." *Amer J Clin Nutr* 100 (2014): 953-958.

219 Tucker, KL, K Moritas, N Qiao, MT Hannan, et al. "Colas, but Not Other Carbonated Beverages, Are Associated with Low Bone Mineral Density in Older Women: the Framingham Osteoporosis Study." *Amer J Clin Nutr* 84 (2006): 936-942.

220 Koek WNH, JB van Muers, BCJ van der Eerden, F Rivadeneira, et al. "The T-13910C Polymorphism in the Lactase Phlorizin Hydrolase Gene Is Associated with Differences in Serum Calcium Levels and Calcium Intake." *J Bone Mineral Res* 25 (2010): 1980-1987.

221 Bacsi, K, JP Kosa,JP, A Lazary, B Balla, et al. "LCT C/T Polymorphism, Serum Calcium and Bone Mineral Density in Postmenopausal Women." *Osteoporosis Intl* 20 (2009): 639-645.

222 Obermayer-Pietsch, BM, CM Bonelli, DE Walter, R Kuhn, et al. "Genetic Predisposition for Adult Lactose Intolerance and Relation to Diet, Bone Density, and Bone Fractures." *J Bone and Mineral Research* 19 (2004): 42-47.

223 Soedamah-Muthu, SS, EL Ding, WK Al-Delaimy, FB Hu, MF Engberink, et al. "Milk and Dairy Consumption and Incidence of Cardiovascular Disease and All-cause Mortality: Dose-Response Meta-Analysis of Prospective Cohort Studies." *Amer J Clin Nutr* 93 (2011): 158-171.

224 Chen, M, Y Li, Q Sun, JE Manson, et al. "Dairy Fat and Risk of Cardiovascular Disease in 3 Cohorts of US Adults." *Amer J Clin Nutr* 104 (2016): 1209-2017.

225 Petruski-Ivleva, N, A Kucharska-Newton, P Palta, D Cooper, et al. "Milk Intake and Cognitive Decline over 20 Years. The Atherosclerosis Risk in Communities (ARIC) Study." *Nutrients* 9:1134 (2017); doi:10.3390/nu9101134.

226 Kesse-Guyot, E, KE Assmann, VA Andreeva, M Ferry, S Hecberg, et al. "Consumption of Dairy Products and Cognitive Functioning: Findings from the SU.VI.MAX 2 Study." *J Nutr and Healthy Aging* 20 (2016): 128-137.

227 O'Connell, S, and G Walsh. "A Novel Acid-stable Acid-active Beta-Galactosidase Potentially Suited to the Alleviation of Lactose Intolerance." *Appl Microbiol Biotechnol* 86 (2010): 517-524.

228 Thompson, WG. Chapter 2, "How the Gut Works," pp. 20-22, in <u>Gut Reactions</u>, Plenum Press, New York, 1989.

229 Turner, KM, G Pasut, and FM Veronese. "Stabilization of a Supplemental Digestive Enzyme by Post-Translational Engineering Using Chemically-Activated Polyethylene Glycol." *Biotechnol Letters* 33 (2011): 617-621.

230 Sheng, Y, H He, and H Zou. "Poly(lactic Acid) Nanoparticles Coated with Combined WGA and Water-Soluble Chitosan for Mucosal Delivery of Beta-Galactosidase." *Drug Delivery* 215 (2014): 370-378.

231 Hoet, PHM, I Bruske-Hohlfeld, and OV Salata. "Nanoparticles – Known and Unknown Health Risks." *J Nanobiotechnology* 2 (2004): 11-16.